American Heart Association®
Learn and Live

Low-Salt
cookbook 4TH EDITION

ALSO BY THE AMERICAN HEART ASSOCIATION

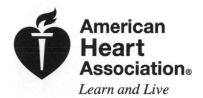

American
Heart
Association®

Learn and Live

Low-Salt
cookbook 4TH EDITION

A COMPLETE GUIDE TO
Reducing Sodium and Fat in Your Diet

HARMONY
BOOKS · NEW YORK

Copyright © 1990, 2001, 2006, 2011 by American Heart Association

No book, including this one, can ever replace the services of a doctor in providing information about your health. You should check with your doctor before using this information in this or any other health-related book.

Published in the United States by Harmony Books, an imprint of the Crown Publishing Group, a division of Penguin Random House LLC, New York.
www.crownpublishing.com

Harmony Books is a trademark and the Circle colophon is a registered trademark of Penguin Random House LLC.

Previous editions of this work were published in the United States by Times Books, New York, in 1990, and by Clarkson Potter/Publishers, an imprint of the Crown Publishing Group, a division of Random House, Inc., New York, in 2001 and 2006.

Your contributions to the American Heart Association support research that helps make publications possible. For more information, call 1-800-AHA-USA1 (1-800-242-8721) or contact us online at www.heart.org.

Library of Congress Cataloging-in-Publication Data
American Heart Association low-salt cookbook : a complete guide to reducing Sodium and fat in your diet.—4th ed.
    p.   cm.
  Includes index.
  1. Salt-free diet—Recipes.   I. American Heart Association.   II. Title: Low-salt Cookbook.
  RM237.8.S73   2011
  641.5'6323—dc22   2010030166

ISBN 978-0-307-58978-1
eISBN 978-0-307-95333-9

Printed in the United States of America

Cover photography by Ben Fink
Cover design by Rae Ann Spitzenberger

10

First Harmony Books Edition

ACKNOWLEDGMENTS

American Heart Association Consumer Publications

DIRECTOR: Linda S. Ball

MANAGING EDITOR: Deborah A. Renza

SENIOR EDITOR: Janice Roth Moss

SCIENCE EDITOR/WRITER: Jacqueline F. Haigney

ASSISTANT EDITOR: Roberta Westcott Sullivan

Recipe Developers

Frank Criscuolo

Nancy S. Hughes

Ruth Mossok Johnston

Jackie Mills, M.S., R.D.

Kathryn Moore

Carol Ritchie

Christy Rost

Julie Shapero, R.D., L.D.

Roxanne Wyss

Nutrition Analyst

Tammi Hancock, R.D.

CONTENTS

PREFACE

For more than 20 years, we have published the *American Heart Association Low-Salt Cookbook* to help people cut back on the salt in their diets. During this time, food preferences and trends in eating habits have changed, and the recipes in this book have evolved along with the tastes of our readers. In this latest volume, you will find heart-healthy, low-sodium dishes from the previous editions plus more than 50 new recipes—including Grilled Flank Steak and Asparagus with Couscous; Carrot, Edamame, and Brown Rice Skillet; and Slow-Cooker Moroccan Chicken—that feature today's most popular ingredients, cooking techniques, and international cuisines.

What hasn't changed is the reason it's so important to limit salt intake: For many people, eating too much sodium can raise blood pressure and even lead to high blood pressure, a disease that has serious consequences if left untreated. High blood pressure increases your risk of developing many health issues, especially cardiovascular problems such as heart disease, heart failure, and stroke. Eating less sodium can help keep your blood pressure low. If you already have high blood pressure, you can often reduce it by eating less salt and making other smart diet and lifestyle changes.

You may believe that if you don't have heart disease or high blood pressure, you don't need to worry about sodium, but that isn't true. According to statistics from the Centers for Disease Control and Prevention, almost 70 percent of all Americans should be eating lower levels of sodium; these people are especially susceptible to the harmful effects of eating too much sodium over time, even if they don't yet have high blood pressure. In fact, by age 50 every American has a 90 percent chance of developing high blood pressure, which, in turn, increases the risk for heart disease and stroke. Given these long-term consequences, reducing the amount of sodium in the food we eat should be a top health priority for most of us.

We understand that it can be a challenge to retrain your taste buds and change long-held habits. As the amount of sodium in the food supply has risen steadily over the years, gradually people have become used to saltier foods. As people eat out more and rely on commercially processed food instead of preparing meals from scratch, they have less control over how much sodium is in their diet. The end result is that many Americans are now eating twice the amount of sodium recommended by the American Heart Association.

The link between a high sodium intake and its negative effects on the circulatory system has been firmly established. In response, federal agencies and the food industry *are* working toward reducing the sodium in processed food while keeping food safe and meeting consumers' expectations for flavor. It may take some time before manufacturers can deliver on all fronts, but, fortunately, you don't have to wait until then to make a dramatic impact on your health. The more you shop smart and cook thoughtfully, the more control you have over your food choices and the amount of sodium you consume. We encourage you to make the *Low-Salt Cookbook* your go-to guide to cut back on sodium while still enjoying the flavors of the foods you eat.

ROSE MARIE ROBERTSON, MD
Chief Science Officer
American Heart Association/American Stroke Association

INTRODUCTION
WELCOME TO A LOW-SALT DIET

Perhaps you've been diagnosed with high blood pressure or have seen it rising over the last few years, maybe you're being proactive about your health because of a family history of high blood pressure, or perhaps your healthcare provider recently told you to start following a low-salt diet to avoid getting high blood pressure or going on medication. Whatever the reason, if you're looking for help on how to reduce the sodium in your diet and thereby manage your blood pressure, you've made an important first step by picking up this book.

SO WHAT'S THE BIG DEAL ABOUT A LITTLE SALT?

The truth of the matter is that most Americans consume *much* more than just a "little" salt and much more than our bodies need. The average person's sodium consumption is 3,400 milligrams a day—more than *double* what is recommended as a healthy level for all adults, regardless of their health status. So, how are we getting so much sodium in our diets? You may be surprised. Here's a breakdown of where most sodium comes from:

- **PROCESSED FOODS:** 77 percent
- **FOODS IN WHICH SODIUM OCCURS NATURALLY** (such as spinach and shrimp): 12 percent
- **SALT ADDED AT THE TABLE:** 6 percent
- **SALT ADDED DURING COOKING:** 5 percent

If, like most other Americans, you consume far too much sodium, you are at a higher risk for high blood pressure. Currently, about one in three American adults has blood pressure above the normal range (prehypertension) and an additional one in three has hypertension, or high blood pressure. Therefore, the American Heart Association now recommends that *everyone* should aim to reduce his or her sodium intake. This means that for maximum health benefit, almost every adult should aim to eat less than 1,500 milligrams (about ⅔ teaspoon) of sodium per day. (This may differ for you if you are directed otherwise by your healthcare provider or you lose a lot of sodium through physical exertion or from heat exposure.)

If you have healthy blood pressure now, the good news is that eating less sodium can help you avoid or delay both prehypertension and hypertension. If you have high blood pressure currently, a low-sodium lifestyle can help you lower it.

Do you love the taste of salt? Even crave it? Believe it or not, you were not born with the desire for salty foods. Salt is actually an acquired taste, and the more salt you eat, the more your taste buds expect it. As a result, food that once might have seemed *too* salty tastes "normal." You can, however, reverse this trend by gradually scaling back on the sodium in your diet and allowing your taste buds to adjust. Be patient, though; it may take more than a month to reduce your desire to salt your food.

CUT THE SALT,
KEEP THE FLAVOR

Although it may seem daunting to try to reduce your sodium intake given the many high-sodium foods on the market and in restaurants today, this book will show you how to gradually and easily make the transition. Fortunately, low sodium does *not* need to mean low flavor! Too much salt can actually mask the subtle flavors of food, so as you get accustomed to using less salt and enjoying the low-sodium recipes in this book, you will experience a wider spectrum of tastes.

The best ways to take control of the sodium in your diet are to learn where to find hidden sodium so you can avoid it and to cook with fewer processed foods, as well as to be mindful of salt-laden food when you eat out. In this cookbook, we offer lots of great ways to do all three—easily and deliciously. In addition to providing you with more than 200 recipes, we'll show you how to:

- **Assess your current eating habits** to understand how the sodium adds up and where you need to make changes (page 6).
- **Develop a personalized eating plan** that provides solid nutrition while helping you control your sodium intake (page 6).
- **Shop wisely to keep sodium low** (pages 14–19), including learning how to read food labels and understanding common packaging terms (pages 20–23).
- **Use healthy cooking techniques** for maximum flavor and benefit without adding salt (pages 26–28), including spicing up foods with a wide variety of salt-free seasonings (pages 24–29).
- **Enjoy eating out without giving in to high-sodium menus** (pages 12–13).

The positive effects of a heart-healthy diet—especially when combined with being regularly physically active and avoiding damaging lifestyle choices such as smoking—are undeniable. To get started, be sure you know your blood pressure numbers. If your blood pressure is still at a healthy level, take action to keep it that way. If it's higher than it should be, changing your diet and getting more regular exercise will both help lower your blood pressure and allow medications to work more effectively. Make today the day you put good lifestyle choices to work for you and your heart, and use the *Low-Salt Cookbook* as your guide to doing just that.

TAKING HEART
Understanding How Sodium Affects Your Health

Your eating habits—especially the amount of sodium you consume—affect your blood pressure and, in turn, your blood pressure affects your heart health. When your blood pressure is higher than it should be, it can damage your circulatory system, causing arteries to thicken and lose elasticity and forcing your heart to work harder. The higher the blood pressure, the greater the risk of heart failure, heart attack, and stroke.

WHAT IS BLOOD PRESSURE?

Blood pressure is the force that blood exerts against the inside of artery walls. It is measured at two different points: when the heart beats (systolic) and when the heart relaxes between beats (diastolic). Blood pressure devices record these pressures in millimeters of mercury (abbreviated as mmHg), and the resulting values are written as systolic over diastolic (for example, 120/80 mmHg). Blood pressure levels are classified as:

- **NORMAL,** when blood pressure is less than 120/80 mmHg.
- **PREHYPERTENSION,** when blood pressure is slightly elevated and falls between the normal and hypertension levels.
- **HYPERTENSION OR HIGH,** when blood pressure is 140/90 mmHg or higher as measured on two separate occasions.

MANAGING YOUR
BLOOD PRESSURE

If you find that your blood pressure is increasing, take action to reduce it *before* it rises to critical levels. High blood pressure usually has no symptoms, so be proactive and keep your blood pressure managed. Here's how:

- **Have your blood pressure checked regularly** (at least once a year, or more if you have high blood pressure).
- **Make smart choices for a healthy diet** by following the American Heart Association dietary recommendations (pages 6–13).
- **Be more physically active** (page 30).
- **Reach and maintain an appropriate body weight** (page 31).
- **Stop smoking and limit alcohol intake** (page 32).
- **Take blood pressure medication as prescribed**, if needed.

These recommendations are the cornerstones of a heart-healthy lifestyle, and making them part of your daily life is the best long-term strategy to keep your blood pumping at healthier levels.

EATING WELL
Following the American Heart Association Dietary Recommendations

To begin your transition to healthier, lower-sodium eating habits, become a savvy sleuth and find out where the sodium in your diet comes from. For one week, write down everything you eat and drink and keep track of the sodium in each item. (See "My Sodium Tracker" on page 320.) Look for sodium values on nutrition labels and on manufacturers' websites; when eating out, check for nutrition information online or at the restaurant. The U.S. Department of Agriculture (USDA) also provides information online. (For more details on reading food labels, see page 20.)

If you're like most other people, as much as three-quarters of the sodium in your diet comes from the salt added during commercial processing. That fact underscores the importance of shopping smart and carefully reading nutrition facts panels, especially because similar products from different manufacturers can contain very different amounts of sodium. When you pay attention to which foods you buy, focus on unprocessed foods, and prepare meals with a minimal amount of added salt, you can significantly reduce the amount of sodium you eat. The more carefully you control the sodium in your diet, the more you are doing to lower your blood pressure or keep it from rising, protect your circulatory system, and prevent heart disease in the future.

INCLUDE A VARIETY OF NUTRIENT-RICH FOODS

To stay healthy, your body requires a variety of foods that supply the full spectrum of nutrients, including fiber, vitamins, and minerals. The American Heart Association eating plan provides all the nutrients you need for optimal health while limiting foods that can put your health at risk. Our guidelines parallel those of the landmark DASH diet (Dietary Approaches to Stop Hypertension), developed by the National Heart, Lung, and Blood Institute. Both eating plans emphasize fruits and vegetables, fiber-rich whole grains, fat-free and low-fat dairy products, fish, lean meats and skinless poultry, legumes, and nuts and seeds.

Many studies have established that you can maintain or lower your blood pressure—even if it's not especially high—by following a healthy eating plan. Including foods rich in potassium can also be important in lowering blood pressure because potassium blunts the effects of sodium. Among the factors that affect blood pressure levels and cardiovascular health are salt intake; the amount and type of fat, cholesterol, protein, and fiber you eat; and your intake of minerals such as potassium, calcium, and magnesium. More than the effect of individual nutrients, however, it is the overall *pattern* of your food choices over time that results in long-term changes in blood pressure and heart health.

As you put together your weekly meal plans, aim to include a variety from all the following food groups. The chart on pages 322–323 shows both how many servings of each food type will offer a good nutritional balance and sample amounts that constitute reasonable portions. The shopping tips on pages 15–19 give you specifics on how to choose foods for the most nutritional payback.

VEGETABLES AND FRUITS. Eating lots of different vegetables and fruits, especially deeply colored ones, will increase the range of nutrients and health benefits these foods provide. Vegetables and fruits are high in vitamins, minerals, and fiber—and in their natural state they are low in calories, which can help you control your weight and therefore help lower or maintain your blood pressure.

FAT-FREE, 1% FAT, AND LOW-FAT DAIRY PRODUCTS. Choose fat-free, 1% fat, and low-fat dairy products, such as milk, yogurt, and cheeses, to get calcium, protein, and other vital nutrients but avoid the saturated fat and cholesterol found in their full-fat or 2% fat counterparts.

FIBER-RICH WHOLE-GRAIN FOODS. Unrefined whole grains are high in both soluble and insoluble fiber, as well as other important nutrients. Eating enough whole grains with fiber can reduce levels of harmful cholesterol and help you feel full, which can make it easier to attain and maintain a healthy body weight. At least half your grain servings should come from whole grains that are rich in fiber.

FISH. Research shows that eating at least two weekly servings of fish, preferably oily fish that contain omega-3 fatty acids (for example, salmon and trout), reduces the risk of heart disease. If you are concerned about the mercury in fish and shellfish, vary the types of fish you eat and remember that levels of mercury depend on the individual fish and the amount eaten. (For up-to-date information on mercury, visit www.USDA.org.) In most cases, the health benefits of eating fish far outweigh the risks.

LEAN MEATS AND SKINLESS POULTRY. To avoid the saturated fat and cholesterol that put your heart health at risk, choose lean and extra-lean cuts of meat and skinless poultry. These foods are excellent sources of protein, as long as you keep portions to a reasonable size. Most adults don't need more than about 6 ounces (cooked weight) of lean poultry and meat each day. (Since meat loses about 25 percent of its weight during cooking,

4 ounces of raw meat will be about 3 ounces cooked.) Instead of thinking of
meat or poultry as the main dish, consider it as a side dish. Try dividing your
plate into four parts: two for vegetables and fruits, one for grains, and the
fourth for a serving of meat, poultry, or other protein source, such as beans.

LEGUMES, NUTS, AND SEEDS. These foods are nutrition power-
houses. Legumes, such as dried beans (although not green beans) and lentils,
are good sources of meatless protein and great sources of fiber. Most nuts and
seeds are nutrient dense, providing protein as well as heart-healthy unsaturated oils. They are also high in calories, however, so eat them in moderation
(a small handful, or about 1½ ounces, is a serving) and without added salt.

UNSATURATED FATS. Fats are an essential part of good nutrition,
and the unsaturated fats found in vegetable oils offer the most health benefit.
Replace butter or stick margarine with unsaturated fats as often as possible,
and use fat-free spray margarines or the light tub margarines that are lowest
in saturated and trans fats. Remember, too, that all fats are high in calories,
so it's important to be aware of how much you use.

LIMIT NUTRIENT-POOR FOODS

An appropriate balance of the nutrient-rich foods just described will give your body what it needs and keep you feeling satisfied. Eating too many nutrient-poor foods, however, just adds calories with little or no nutritional value, leaving less room for more nutritious foods. In many cases, nutrient-poor foods also contain high levels of sodium, added sugars, and harmful fats. For your overall good health, limit your intake of foods that fall into the following categories.

FOODS HIGH IN SODIUM. Although sodium is vital in maintaining the complicated balance of fluids and electrolytes in your body, it's easy to consume more of it than you realize, especially when eating processed or restaurant foods. Get in the habit of checking the sodium content of foods you buy or eat away from home. Work toward lowering your sodium intake, starting by eating less than 2,300 milligrams per day. For the greatest health benefit, aim for less than 1,500 milligrams per day. (For a list of foods that are particularly high in sodium, see pages 324–325.)

HIGH-CALORIE, LOW-NUTRIENT FOODS AND BEVERAGES. Eating a lot of added sugars can lead to weight gain, which in turn makes developing high blood pressure more likely; being over-weight and having high blood pressure both increase the risk of heart disease. "Added sugars" means sugars and syrups that are added to foods during processing, preparation, or at the table. Common sources of added sugars include regular soft drinks, fruit drinks, sweetened milk products, sweetened snacks and desserts, and candy. Limit high-calorie beverages such as sugar-sweetened sodas and fruit drinks; keep in mind that one 12-ounce can of regular soda contains about 8 teaspoons of added sugar and no nutritional value. Save high-calorie snacks and desserts for occasional treats rather than everyday choices.

FOODS HIGH IN SATURATED AND TRANS FATS. A steady diet of foods rich in saturated and trans fats raises your risk of heart disease by increasing the amount of harmful cholesterol that circulates in your bloodstream. Saturated fats come from animal-based foods, such as meat, poultry, whole-milk dairy products (cream, butter, and cheese, for example), and lard, as well as from certain tropical vegetable oils (coconut, palm, and palm kernel). Choosing lean and extra-lean cuts of meat and skinless poultry and replacing whole-fat and 2% dairy products with fat-free, 1% fat, and low-fat alternatives will help you keep your intake of saturated fat low (less than 7 percent of your total daily calories). Trans fat is found in many commercial food products as a result of hydrogenation, the processing that makes liquid oils more solid. Examples of these products include baked goods, fried foods, snack foods, vegetable shortening, stick margarine, and other foods made with partially hydrogenated vegetable oils. Manufacturers and restaurants are constantly reformulating their products to reduce or eliminate trans fat, however, so continue to check for updated nutrition information. Aim to eat as little trans fat as possible (less than 1 percent of your total daily calories).

FOODS HIGH IN CHOLESTEROL. Dietary cholesterol also may contribute to the level of harmful cholesterol in your blood, so aim for an intake of less than 300 milligrams each day. Remember that dietary cholesterol comes only from animal products; vegetable-based foods do not contain cholesterol. The foods that contain the most cholesterol include egg yolks, whole milk, full-fat cheese, animal fats, organ meats, and some types of shellfish, such as shrimp and crayfish.

CHOOSE WELL
WHEN DINING OUT

Americans are eating in restaurants and getting takeout meals more than ever, and the food is typically highly salted. Although watching your sodium intake can be a challenge away from home, don't let it spoil the pleasure of dining out. Just follow the same basic principles when you decide what to order as you would at home.

Many chain restaurants now provide nutrition information for their menu items. To see how much you can decrease the sodium you are eating when you dine out, compare the sodium values for your favorite menu choices with some lower-sodium alternatives. As a rule of thumb, the less preparation a food item undergoes, the less sodium it will contain.

DINE-IN RESTAURANTS. When ordering, be as specific as you can about what you want and how you want it prepared. If possible, ask to have your dish made without salt, and get sauces and dressings on the side so you can control how much you eat. Choose foods that are grilled, steamed, or baked instead of fried, and try to avoid dishes that contain a lot of cheese or other high-sodium dairy products.

FAST FOOD. The same strategies for dine-in apply to fast-food restaurants. Reading nutrition information and educating yourself about what you are ordering is especially important for fast-food options, which are usually high in sodium, saturated fat, trans fat, cholesterol, *and* calories. Go online or ask in the restaurant for the nutrition information for your favorite foods. Be prepared: Make comparisons and decide in advance which are the healthiest options so you'll know what to order even when you're in a hurry. Remember that depending on the dressing and other ingredients you choose, salads can be as high in sodium and calories as a burger. Avoid high-sodium cheese and condiments such as ketchup, mustard, soy sauce, salad dressing, pickles, and olives. Beware of "special" sauces unless you know what they contain.

When you find yourself ordering food that you know doesn't fit into your eating plan, think *small*! Portion control is an effective way to cut down on excess sodium, as well as calories, saturated and trans fats, and cholesterol. For example, have just one slice of vegetable pizza or choose a small burger with lettuce, tomato, and onion—without cheese. Split an entrée with a friend or plan to take half home. You can also compensate for high-sodium restaurant meals by choosing very low sodium foods later that day or on the next. By staying aware of what you're eating and following a few simple rules, you'll be able to enjoy eating out without jeopardizing your health.

FIVE EASY STEPS TO EATING WELL
To turn awareness into action, start with these simple steps.

1. **Introduce changes at a gradual pace.** If you now eat one or two vegetables a day, try to add a serving at dinner every day for a week. The next week, add a serving at lunch as well.
2. **Increase the proportion of vegetables to meat in your meals.** Fill your plate with lots of different vegetable dishes. Use extra vegetables in stir-fries and casseroles, and add grated vegetables to ground beef before shaping it into hamburgers and meat loaf.
3. **Include two or more meat-free meals each week.** Replace meats with alternatives such as dried beans and other legumes, and incorporate vegetable-based meat substitutes, such as tofu and soy crumbles, into your favorite recipes.
4. **Replace high-sodium, high-calorie snacks with healthier choices.** To make your own snacks, try the recipes in "Appetizers & Snacks" on pages 37–48. In general, choose a variety of fruits and vegetables as well as fat-free or low-fat dairy products and fiber-rich whole-grain foods.
5. **Decrease the added sugars in your diet.** Replace sugar-sweetened beverages, such as regular sodas and fruit drinks, with water or fat-free or low-fat (1%) milk and fruit smoothies, and use sweets as special-occasional treats.

SHOPPING SAVVY
Knowing What to Look for in the Grocery Store

One of the keys to eating well is to shop smart. Because so much of the sodium in the food supply comes from processed and prepared foods, the grocery store is really the place to start cutting back. When you're making your selections, remember to check nutrition labels for sodium as well as calories, saturated and trans fats, and cholesterol. It's a good idea to research online which foods are manufactured in low-sodium versions, since some are not widely available. If your store doesn't stock the low-sodium foods you need, ask the manager to order them.

FILL YOUR CART
WITH HEALTHY FOODS

Each type of healthy food contributes in its own way to a complete and balanced diet. Knowing what to look for and how to make the best choices are important parts of being a smart shopper. Here are some helpful shopping strategies:

- Start by focusing on the foods located around the perimeter of the store—that's usually where you'll find the fresh produce, dairy products, seafood, poultry, and meats.
- Next, choose your grains, legumes, nuts, and oils to round our your selections.
- Finally, add some carefully chosen packaged foods and beverages.

The idea is to base the larger part of your diet on the major food groups to maximize nutritional value.

VEGETABLES AND FRUITS. Fill your shopping cart with your favorites, and experiment with new choices so you don't get into a rut. When buying produce, choose deeply colored vegetables and fruits. While in the produce aisle, visualize a rainbow and choose a fruit or vegetable that represents each color to help ensure that you get a variety. Some good choices are:

- **GREEN:** arugula, broccoli, spinach, kiwifruit
- **RED:** tomatoes, red bell peppers, apples, strawberries
- **YELLOW:** bananas, yellow bell peppers, apples, summer squash
- **ORANGE:** sweet potatoes, carrots, cantaloupe
- **PURPLE/BLUE:** eggplant, plums, blueberries

When you're buying frozen or canned vegetables and fruits, always read the package labels, and shop for products that are not processed with salt, added sugars, or saturated and trans fats. One-half cup of fruit juice or low-sodium vegetable juice counts as one serving, but to get the advantage of fiber, it's best to eat the whole fruit or vegetable.

DAIRY PRODUCTS. If you use full-fat milk now, gradually transition to 2% fat milk, then to 1%, and finally to fat-free as your taste buds adjust. In addition to fat-free milk, look for fat-free and low-fat versions of yogurt, sour cream, cream cheese, half-and-half, ice cream, and many varieties of cheese, such as Cheddar, mozzarella, American, and Swiss. With the exception of buttermilk and cheese, most milk products do not contain added salt, but you should read labels as you make your choices.

FIBER-RICH WHOLE GRAINS. Look for breads, cereals, pastas, and other foods that list a whole grain as the first ingredient on the nutrition label. Breads are typically high in sodium, but products vary widely, so be sure to check the nutrition facts panels before you buy. Try different kinds of bread, such as whole or cracked wheat, whole-grain rye, and whole-grain oat. Look for "light" bread and thinner or smaller slices, which usually contain less sodium. Buy whole-grain crackers that are lower in sodium, such as Scandinavian-style crispbreads, instead of heavily seasoned snack crackers.

Most plain cooked cereals, rices, and pastas are good choices if you don't add salt to the cooking water. (Remember to read nutrition labels and ingredient lists to check for added salt.) When choosing rice, try to use brown rice instead of white, which has had the nutritive germ and bran removed. Try less-familiar grains, such as quinoa, barley, amaranth, and farro. With pastas, be especially careful which sauces you add. Most manufactured spaghetti sauces are very high in sodium, so be sure to compare different products. Making your own sauce (page 264) is an easy way to enjoy your favorite pastas without added salt.

Limit your use of prepared mixes and commercial baked goods, such as muffins, biscuits, rolls, cakes, and cookies. Even if they contain some whole grain, these products usually also contain significant amounts of sodium, as well as saturated fat, trans fat, cholesterol, and added sugars. Instead, bake your own healthy versions. Use the recipes in this book, or omit the salt from your favorite recipes and use the ingredient substitutions listed on page 329.

FISH. When choosing fish, put the emphasis on those that are high in omega-3 fatty acids. Such fish include salmon, tuna, trout, herring, and mackerel. Whether you use fresh or frozen fish, it is easy and quick to prepare (you can thaw frozen fish in a few minutes by soaking the packages in cold water). Another option is canned very low sodium albacore or light tuna packed in water. Most shellfish are high in protein and very low in saturated fat, but some, such as shrimp, are naturally higher in sodium and cholesterol. You can still enjoy them as part of a healthy eating plan; just remember to stay within the recommended guidelines.

POULTRY AND MEATS. Remember that skinless white-meat poultry is lower in saturated fat than the dark meat. If you buy poultry with skin, remove the skin before eating the meat. Stay away from self-basting and brined poultry because the broth used is usually high in sodium and saturated fat. Look for lean cuts of beef, such as round steak, sirloin tip, tenderloin, and extra-lean ground beef, or pork, including tenderloin, loin chops, and low-sodium center-cut ham. Whether you buy poultry, beef, or pork, be sure to discard all the fat you see. In general, canned, processed, and deli meats, such as frankfurters, sausage, corned beef, salt pork, and smoked or dried meats (including ham and bacon), are high in sodium, saturated fat, and cholesterol, so limit these foods to very occasional uses.

LEGUMES, NUTS, AND SEEDS. Legumes, such as dried beans, lentils, peas, edamame (green soybeans), and peanuts, are rich in fiber and provide plenty of protein. To take advantage of the nutritional benefits of legumes, use them as the base of meatless meals. Keep no-salt-added canned beans on hand for easy entrées and to add to side-dish soups and salads. Unsalted nuts and seeds are good sources of potassium, magnesium, fiber, and protein. Buy them to use as snacks or to add to salads or muffins, for example.

FATS AND OILS. The primary types of fat found in food are saturated and unsaturated. You can tell the difference when shopping because unsaturated fats and oils stay liquid at room temperature, whereas saturated fats, such as butter, tend to stay hard. (Trans fat results from hydrogenation, the commercial processing used to make liquid fats more solid, as in stick margarines, for example.) Heart-healthy unsaturated fats may be either polyunsaturated or monounsaturated, and most oils contain a combination of these fats in varying percentages. Canola, corn, olive, safflower, soybean, and sunflower oils are all good choices; they contain no sodium and are cholesterol free and low in saturated fat. Use these oils, nonstick cooking sprays, and light tub margarine to replace stick margarine, butter, and shortening. When buying prepared salad dressings, be sure to check labels; most commercial salad dressings contain large amounts of sodium. You can drastically cut the sodium by making your own dressings using the recipes on pages 95–100.

BEVERAGES AND SNACKS. When you're thirsty, reach for water (try flavoring it with lemon, lime, or orange wedges), fat-free milk, and other unsweetened drink choices. Think of sugary sodas and other sugar-sweetened drinks as occasional treats rather than as accompaniments to a meal. Some diet soft drinks, sports and energy drinks, and mineral waters are high in sodium. Just as you check when you buy food, be sure to check the nutrition labels on beverages as well. (If you're trying to keep your sodium intake very low, check on the sodium content of your local water supply through your town's utility department. The level of sodium in tap water varies widely from one location to another, and in some areas the water is softened with added sodium. If your tap water is especially high in sodium, you may want to switch to low-sodium bottled water for drinking.)

When you do buy commercial snack foods, choose products with the least amount of sodium, saturated and trans fats, and empty calories from added sugars. It's important to read labels carefully: Manufacturers are working to reformulate their products to eliminate the trans fat in partially hydrogenated oils, but in some cases the trans fat is replaced with large amounts of saturated fat. Instead, try good-for-you snacks, such as Baked Veggie Chips (page 46), air-popped popcorn, dried fruit, frozen grapes, and unsalted nuts. Ingredients are shown on packaging in order of volume, so avoid foods that list sugar, sucrose, glucose, fructose, maltose, dextrose, corn syrup, high-fructose corn syrup, concentrated fruit juice, or honey at or near the beginning of the ingredient list.

CONDIMENTS AND SEASONINGS. Many of your favorite condiments may add more sodium to your meals than you realize. Favorites such as ketchup, mustard, and, especially, soy sauce can turn low-salt foods into sodium bombs. Many of these familiar items are also available in no-salt or low-salt varieties, however. New and reformulated products come out all the time, so watch store shelves for them and check labels regularly. You can also look for no-salt-added products online, in the special-foods area of your store, or in health-food stores. The products listed below can "secretly" but significantly increase salt content, so shop for the no-salt-added or low-sodium varieties.

- Commercial soups and bouillon cubes
- Salad dressings
- Relishes and pickles
- Ketchup and mustards
- Sauces such as soy, Worcestershire, barbecue, steak, and chili
- Flavored seasoning salts

Be aware that herb and spice blends and other seasonings may contain salt. Check the ingredients to see whether "salt," "sodium," or any related words (such as "monosodium glutamate," or MSG) are listed. As you might expect, any seasoning product that uses "salt" as part of the name is high in sodium; common examples are onion salt, garlic salt, and celery salt.

If you're considering buying a salt substitute, be sure to read the labels. Many salt substitutes contain a large amount of potassium and very little sodium; most people can use them freely, but not people who have certain health conditions (kidney disease, for example) or take medications that cause the body to retain potassium. Talk with your healthcare professional about whether a salt substitute is a good option for you.

To keep sodium very low, make your own versions of the common sauces, condiments, and seasonings with recipes on pages 259–278. For example, foods packed in brine, such as pickles, are loaded with sodium; making your own pickles, such as Sweet Bread-and-Butter Pickles (page 274), is simple and much healthier. For brined foods that you aren't likely to make for yourself—olives and capers are examples—limit your quantities.

READ NUTRITION INFORMATION AND FOOD ICONS

When you buy fresh produce and other unprocessed foods, you have total control over how much fat, salt, and extra calories you add. With packaged or prepared foods, however, the only way to be sure of what you're getting is to check the nutrition facts panel. The U.S. Food and Drug Administration (FDA) and the USDA regulate the information on the panel to help you compare products and understand what you are buying. Other organizations, including the American Heart Association (see page 23), use their own icon systems to help you make decisions, and some grocery stores have introduced on-shelf labeling programs. When you see an icon or wording that signals a health claim on the front of food packaging, evaluate the nutrition facts panel and the ingredient list before you make your selections.

HOW TO READ THE NUTRITION FACTS PANEL. Pay attention to the serving size as it relates to the nutrient numbers. A container may look like it holds one serving, but the numbers on the panel may have been calculated for more. If, for example, the panel says the container holds two servings and you intend to eat the entire contents, you must double all the values given and consider how they will add to your overall intake of calories, sodium, saturated fat, trans fat, and cholesterol. Keep in mind that for a 2,000-calorie diet, 40 calories (2% or less) per serving is considered low, 100 calories (5% or less) per serving is considered moderate, and 400 calories (40%) or more per serving is considered high.

The % Daily Value column tells you the percentage of each nutrient in a single serving, in terms of the daily recommended amount. As a guide, if you want to consume less of a nutrient, such as sodium, saturated fat, trans fat, or cholesterol, choose foods with a lower % Daily Value (5% or less is considered low). If you want to consume more of a nutrient, such as fiber, look for foods with a higher % Daily Value (20% or more is considered high).

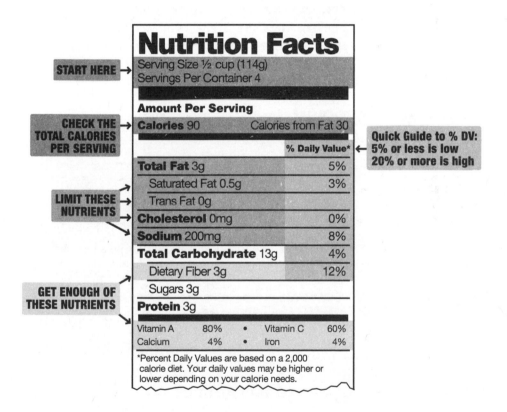

Nutrition Facts

START HERE → Serving Size ½ cup (114g)
Servings Per Container 4

Amount Per Serving

CHECK THE → Calories 90   Calories from Fat 30
TOTAL CALORIES PER SERVING

                               % Daily Value*

Quick Guide to % DV:
← 5% or less is low
20% or more is high

Total Fat 3g	**5%**
Saturated Fat 0.5g	**3%**
Trans Fat 0g	
Cholesterol 0mg	**0%**
Sodium 200mg	**8%**
Total Carbohydrate 13g	**4%**
Dietary Fiber 3g	**12%**
Sugars 3g	
Protein 3g	

LIMIT THESE NUTRIENTS →

GET ENOUGH OF THESE NUTRIENTS →

Vitamin A	80%	•	Vitamin C	60%
Calcium	4%	•	Iron	4%

*Percent Daily Values are based on a 2,000 calorie diet. Your daily values may be higher or lower depending on your calorie needs.

Some foods contain added sodium compounds, which are noted in ingredient lists. Common examples include *sodium alginate* (used in many chocolate milks and ice creams to make a smooth mixture); *sodium benzoate* (used as a preservative in many condiments, such as relishes, sauces, and salad dressings); *sodium hydroxide* (used in food processing to soften and loosen skins of ripe olives and certain fruits and vegetables); *sodium nitrite* (used in cured meats and sausages); *sodium propionate* (used in pasteurized cheese and in some breads and cakes to inhibit the growth of molds); and *sodium sulfite* (used to bleach certain fruits, such as maraschino cherries and glazed or crystallized fruits, that are to be artificially colored; also used as a preservative in some dried fruits, such as prunes).

SORTING OUT SODIUM. Food labels use certain names or phrases to describe the sodium content of the food. Each has a meaning defined by the FDA and the USDA. Knowing what each means can help you make the best choice.

- **"SODIUM FREE"** means 5 mg sodium or less per serving.
- **"VERY LOW SODIUM"** means 35 mg sodium or less per serving.
- **"LOW SODIUM"** means 140 mg sodium or less per serving.
- **"REDUCED SODIUM"** means at least 25% less sodium than in the original version. (Be aware, however, that many reduced-sodium foods, such as chicken broth, soups, and soy sauce, still contain a significant amount of sodium.)
- **"UNSALTED" OR "NO SALT ADDED"** means no salt was added during processing. (This does not necessarily mean, however, that this product is sodium free.)

These terms refer only to sodium content; it's important to read labels carefully since some foods that have little if any sodium may be high in saturated or trans fats, calories, or cholesterol.

AMERICAN HEART ASSOCIATION FOOD CERTIFICATION PROGRAM. The American Heart Association's heart-check mark helps you quickly and reliably find heart-healthy foods in the grocery store. When you see the heart-check mark on food packaging, you know that the food has been certified by the association to meet our criteria for saturated fat and cholesterol. To learn more about how you can use the heart-check mark when you shop, visit www.heartcheckmark.org.

Low in Saturated Fat & Cholesterol

CERTIFIED by
American Heart Association
heartcheckmark.org

COOKING SMART
Preparing Healthy Meals

Get started by thinking in terms of seasoning for flavor, not for the taste of salt. Experiment on your own with new combinations of spices and herbs and take advantage of low-sodium stocks, all-fruit juices, and table wines to deepen and enrich the range of flavors in your favorite dishes. Our recipes also show you how to make your own heart-healthy versions of foods and condiments that are typically high in sodium, such as soups and broths, breads, sauces, and seasonings.

KEEP THE FLAVOR
WITHOUT THE SALT

When you're cooking at home, you'll want to use plenty of pepper, garlic, onion, and/or lemon to give foods more distinctive flavor. Instead of onion salt, garlic salt, and celery salt, switch to onion powder, garlic powder, and celery seeds or flakes, which are all low in sodium and provide lots of impact. Replace salt with herbs and spices or a salt-free seasoning mix, or get creative and prepare your own salt-free seasoning blends.

You can also refer to Ingredient Substitutions on page 329 for ideas about how to reduce the sodium and harmful fat in the recipes you love. For example, to tenderize meats, marinate them rather than using high-sodium meat tenderizer. Instead of using seasoned bread crumbs, add salt-free herbs to unseasoned bread crumbs. Make these and the following expert tips part of your kitchen repertoire to satisfy your taste buds while using less salt in your food.

- **Add fresh herbs to dishes** at the last minute for a more "alive" taste. In most recipes, fresh herbs provide more flavor than dried.
- **Buy the best and the freshest whole spices** and grind them in a spice grinder. You'll taste a big difference compared to preground dried spices.
- **If you do buy preground dried spices or herbs,** purchase only small amounts. You'll need to replenish your supply more often, but they'll be fresher.
- **Use dry mustard or no-salt-added bottled mustard** instead of high-sodium bottled mustard. You can also try honey mustard, which is generally lower in sodium than other bottled mustards. Check the nutrition labels when new products appear; some are low in sodium without advertising it on the front.

- **Add fresh hot chile peppers to your dishes for a little bite.** (Using plastic gloves, discard the seeds and ribs before finely chopping the peppers if you like less heat.) Raw peppers are very low in sodium and have a lot more flavor than the higher-sodium pickled kind.

- **Use a food processor to grate fresh horseradish,** which packs more punch than the salted, bottled kind.

- **Add fresh gingerroot for a lot of zing.** Peel the gingerroot, then grate it using a ginger grater, microplane grater, or flat, sheet-type grater.

- **Grate citrus zest,** the part of the peel without the bitter white pith, with either a microplane grater or a flat, sheet-type grater. You can also remove the zest with a vegetable peeler and cut it into thin strips.

- **Try sprinkling vinegar or citrus juice on foods to enhance flavor,** but add it at the last minute. Vinegar is wonderful on vegetables such as greens; citrus juice, on fruits such as cantaloupe.

- **Stay away from cooking wines and sherries;** they are very high in sodium. Although you don't need to use an expensive selection, the wine you cook with should taste good enough to drink.

- **Fill a salt or pepper shaker with a combination of finely ground dried herbs and spices** to use instead of salt, or buy salt-free herb blends.

- **Some vegetables and fruits,** such as mushrooms, tomatoes, chiles, cherries, cranberries, and currants, impart a more intense flavor when dried than when fresh. When you reconstitute them, the soaking liquid will give you a bonus of natural "broth" to work with.

- **Dry-roast seeds, nuts, and whole spices to bring out their full flavor.** See the Cook's Tip on page 40 for instructions.

USE HEART-HEALTHY
COOKING TECHNIQUES

All cooking methods are not created equal: Some are better than others for preserving basic nutrients and keeping added fat and sodium to a minimum. Try to avoid methods that add fat or allow food to cook in its own fat, such as deep-fat frying or pan frying. Instead, use the following techniques to enhance flavor and help protect your heart.

BRAISING OR STEWING. Both of these slow-cooking methods are good ways to tenderize tougher cuts of meat. They both involve covering and cooking food in liquid. To braise food, add only a small amount of liquid to the pot. To stew, add enough liquid to cover the ingredients. Because fat cooks out of the meat into the liquid, prepare your recipe a day ahead, if possible. Refrigerate the dish so you can then easily remove the chilled fat before reheating the food. Braising and stewing are also excellent ways to cook vegetables and fruit.

GRILLING OR BROILING. Grilling (cooking over direct heat) and broiling (cooking under direct heat) allow the fat to drip away from food as it cooks. These methods are best for foods that cook quickly, such as steaks, chicken pieces, seafood, and vegetables. For extra flavor, marinate food before putting it on the grill or under the broiler and baste during the cooking process. (For food safety, be sure to clean basting brushes between steps to prevent transferring bacteria from raw meat.)

MICROWAVE COOKING. Microwaving is a fast, easy method that keeps food moist as it cooks. Because microwaving does not cause the liquid in food to evaporate, you need no added fat or oil to prevent sticking. Microwaving is particularly useful for foods that cook well in moist heat, such as fish, poultry, vegetables, and soups. To convert regular recipes for microwaving, try cutting the cooking time to one-fourth or one-third; test the food and continue cooking for short periods until it reaches the desired doneness. Microwaves vary in power, so follow your manufacturer's timing instructions. If you are adapting a recipe for the microwave, remember to reduce the liquid used by about one-third and to keep food pieces similar in size so they will cook evenly.

POACHING. To poach a food, typically chicken or fish, immerse it in a pan of just-simmering liquid on top of the stove. Liquids commonly used include wine, water, and fat-free, low-sodium broths. After you poach the food, remove it and, if using a cooking liquid other than water, rapidly boil the liquid to reduce it to a sauce.

SLOW COOKING. Slow cookers can make it easy to have a home-cooked dinner waiting at the end of a busy day. Be sure to layer the ingredients as the recipe directs, because foods cook faster at the bottom of the cooker. Cover the cooker and cook on low or high, as directed. Unless the recipe says otherwise, it's best not to uncover or stir the contents while they cook because you'll let out heat and moisture.

STEAMING. Steam food by placing it in a steamer basket over simmering water in a tightly covered saucepan or skillet. Especially good for vegetables, steaming leaves the natural flavor, color, and nutritional value of food intact. Any food that can be simmered or boiled can be steamed. Try adding herbs to the water or using low-sodium broth, wine, or fruit juice instead of water to add even more flavor to the finished dish.

STIR-FRYING. The high temperature and the constant movement of stir-frying in a small amount of hot oil preserves the color and crispness of vegetables and seals in the juices of meats, poultry, and seafood as they cook. Traditionally, stir-frying is done in a wok with sloping sides, but a large skillet will also work well. Take the time to prep ingredients and measure out sauces before you start to cook, because stir-frying goes quickly once begun. Many stir-fry recipes call for soy sauce, which is usually very high in sodium. Read labels and choose the lowest-sodium version available.

ROASTING AND BAKING. Roasting and baking use dry heat to cook foods. For roasting poultry and meats, trim and discard all visible fat and place the food on a rack; that will keep the food from sitting in fat drippings while it cooks. Baste with low-sodium, fat-free liquids, such as broth, wine, no-salt-added tomato juice, or fresh lemon juice, to keep the food moist. Test for doneness with an instant-read thermometer inserted into the thickest part of the meat but not touching bone. Because roasting caramelizes their natural sugars, it is also excellent for cooking many types of vegetables. For baking, which usually uses lower temperatures than roasting, you don't need a rack. Follow the recipe directions for whether to cover the pot. Poultry, seafood, and meat dishes can be baked in covered cookware with a little liquid to add flavor and keep food moist; casseroles, breads, and many desserts also call for baking.

HEART-HEALTHY
COOKING TIPS

Use these techniques to cut back on calories, saturated fat, and cholesterol— as well as sodium.

- **Always use the lowest-sodium products available.** These may be labeled "sodium-free," "salt-free," "no-salt-added," "very-low sodium," or "low-sodium." The difference between these products and their "regular" counterparts can be very significant.

- **Use a nonstick skillet** so you can cook foods with a minimum of oil, or use cooking spray. (Check the warranty information from your cookware's manufacturer. Some recommend against using cooking spray on nonstick surfaces.)

- **Trim away and discard all visible fat** from meat before cooking. For poultry, remove the fat and skin, except when roasting whole poultry. (Discard the cooked skin before eating the poultry.) Raw skin will be easier to remove if you use paper towels or a clean cloth to take hold of it. To help prevent the spread of bacteria, scrub the cutting surface and utensils well with hot, sudsy water after preparing meat or poultry.

- **After you roast meat or poultry, chill the drippings in the refrigerator.** Once the drippings are cooled, the fat will rise to the top and harden. You can then remove it easily and save the liquid to use in stews, sauces, and soups.

- **Use more fruit and vegetables in unexpected places.** Try adding chopped broccoli as a "hidden" layer in your next lasagna, or include shredded zucchini in meat loaf, pumpkin in this weekend's batch of pancakes, or berries or orange wedges in tonight's green salad. Be creative! Adding finely chopped vegetables is also a great way to stretch ground poultry or meat to feed more people.

- **Try using fat-free, low-sodium broth instead of water** to cook rice and other grains for richer flavor.

- **Seal in natural juices by wrapping foods in aluminum foil** or cooking parchment before cooking. Or try wrapping foods in edible pouches made of large steamed lettuce or cabbage leaves and baking them with the seam side down.

- **Make your own salad dressing** so you can control the amounts of sodium and calories on your greens. Prepare enough to keep on hand in the refrigerator for the same convenience you get from commercial bottled dressings.

In addition to following a heart-healthy eating plan, making wise lifestyle choices is essential to good health. It's always important to stay physically active, maintain a healthy weight, and eliminate the habits that put your heart at risk, especially if you are concerned about your blood pressure.

MAKE PHYSICAL ACTIVITY PART OF YOUR ROUTINE

Being physically active is crucial to maintaining your weight, energy, and overall health, and the lasting benefits are huge. Exercising daily can prevent blood pressure from rising as you get older. If you already have high blood pressure, being physically active will help lower it, increase the effectiveness of blood pressure medications, and decrease your risk for heart disease and stroke.

Aerobic exercises, such as brisk walking, jogging, swimming, and biking, directly benefit your heart. You should aim for at least 150 minutes (2 hours and 30 minutes) of moderate-intensity, or 75 minutes (1 hour and 15 minutes) of vigorous-intensity, aerobic exercise each week. Moderate-intensity activities increase your heart rate to the point that you are able to talk but not sing while you are exercising. At vigorous intensity, you should not be able to say more than a few words without needing to catch your breath. You can combine activities at different intensities, and you can also break your workout time into sessions of 10 minutes or more, spread out through the week, to reach an equivalent total. Twice a week or more, you should also include moderate- or high-intensity muscle-strengthening activities that involve all the major muscle groups.

REACH AND MAINTAIN
A HEALTHY WEIGHT

Being overweight or obese is a major risk factor for diabetes and cardiovascular disease, especially high blood pressure. People who are overweight or obese are much more likely to have high blood pressure than those at a healthy weight. When you are overweight or obese, your body needs more energy to carry more weight. To provide that energy, your heart must work harder. Over time, the heavier workload causes the heart to enlarge and weaken.

If you are overweight or obese, losing weight can help you lower your blood pressure and blood cholesterol levels. For many overweight people, losing just 10 percent of their body weight can reduce blood pressure or prevent high blood pressure. Although the American Heart Association dietary recommendations are not intended as a weight-loss plan, they emphasize nutritious foods such as fruits and vegetables that are low in calories and fiber-rich whole grains that can help you feel full. Despite the claims of fad diets, the key to losing weight is logical and simple: eat fewer calories and increase your level of physical activity. To start an effective weight-loss program, you need to know your recommended calorie intake. Compare that with the number of calories you are actually eating and the number of calories you are burning through physical activity to see how much you need to cut back. (For more information on determining your calorie intake and healthy weight loss, visit www.heart.org.)

A gradual weight loss of about 1 to 2 pounds per week is best. It's a safe approach, and if you stick to that goal, you'll be more likely to keep the pounds off for the long term. To cut calories, add a routine of aerobic physical activity and eat smaller portions, substitute lower-calorie foods for high-calorie ones, follow a set weight-loss diet plan, or combine all these techniques. Talk with your healthcare provider to decide which approach is best for you.

STOP SMOKING AND
LIMIT ALCOHOL INTAKE

Smoking increases blood pressure, decreases your ability to exercise, and increases the tendency of blood to clot. If you smoke now, find a way to quit. Family and friends, support groups, and your healthcare professional can help you find a program that will work for you. Regardless of how long you have been a smoker, your risk of heart disease and stroke will begin to drop dramatically as soon as you beat the habit.

Although some studies have shown health benefits from drinking moderate amounts of alcohol, research also consistently shows that people who drink more than moderate levels tend to develop high blood pressure. Alcohol is a major source of calories and can contribute to weight gain, which in turn can further increase blood pressure. A moderate amount means no more than two drinks per day for a man and no more than one drink per day for a woman. One drink is 12 ounces of beer, 4 ounces of wine, or 1½ ounces of 80-proof hard liquor. If you don't drink alcohol now, don't start; if you drink more than is considered moderate, find ways to cut back.

RECIPES

To help you keep track of what you are eating, every recipe in this cookbook includes a panel of nutrition information. We make every effort to ensure that the nutrition analyses are accurate and up-to-date, but because of the many variables involved, the data should be considered approximate.

ABOUT THE NUTRITION ANALYSES

- **Each analysis is based on a single serving** unless otherwise indicated; optional ingredients or garnishes are not analyzed.
- **When figuring portions,** remember that the measured amounts given for serving sizes are approximate.
- **All the recipes are analyzed using unsalted or low-sodium ingredients** whenever possible. If this book provides a recipe for a common ingredient—for example, chicken broth—we use the data for our own version in the analysis. If only a regular commercial product is available, we use the one with the least sodium.
- **Values other than fats** are rounded to the nearest whole number. Fat values are rounded to the nearest half gram. Because of the rounding, values for saturated, trans, monounsaturated, and polyunsaturated fats may not add up to the amount shown for total fat value.
- **When a recipe lists ingredient options,** we analyze the first one.
- **Ingredients with a range**—for example, a 2½- to 3-pound chicken—are analyzed using the average of the range.

- **Meats are analyzed as cooked and lean,** with all visible fat discarded. Values for ground beef are based on extra-lean meat that is 95 percent fat free.
- **If meat, poultry, or seafood is marinated** and the marinade is discarded, we calculate only the amount of marinade absorbed.
- **We specify canola, corn, and olive oils** in these recipes, but you can also use other heart-healthy unsaturated oils, such as safflower, soybean, and sunflower.
- **If a recipe calls for alcohol,** we estimate that most of the alcohol calories evaporate during the cooking process.
- **Because product labeling in the marketplace can vary** and change quickly, we use the generic terms "fat-free" and "low-fat" throughout to avoid confusion.
- **We use the abbreviations** "g" for gram and "mg" for milligram.

EXPERIMENT AND ENJOY

Although specific ingredients are listed for each recipe, we encourage you to experiment as you cook. As long as you don't use an ingredient that adds sodium or any of the other dietary villains, changing herbs, spices, spirits, vinegars, and vegetables will give you variety and allow you to customize the recipe to your taste. Whether you choose fresh or dried herbs or fresh, bottled, or frozen citrus juices will not affect the nutrition analysis, but fresh will usually taste best, especially in uncooked dishes.

Also, check the index for the Cook's Tips that are scattered throughout the recipe pages and discuss interesting ingredients and techniques. Finally, refer to "Ingredients Substitutions" (page 329) and "Emergency Substitutions" (pages 330–331) to learn how to adapt your favorite recipes or make do when you're out of an ingredient that you need.

SPECIAL DIET INSTRUCTIONS

If your healthcare provider or dietitian has given you specific instructions for a prescribed low-sodium diet, check its requirements against the ingredients used in these recipes. In case of a difference, be sure to follow the advice of your healthcare provider. If, for example, your instructions specify to eat only unsalted bread, use that in place of the regular bread listed in our recipes. (Remember that such substitutions will change the nutritional content from the analysis listed with each recipe.)

APPETIZERS & SNACKS

EDAMAME-AVOCADO DIP

This vibrant green dip is perfect for serving with fresh vegetables. You can make it up to three days in advance and refrigerate it in an airtight container—the lime juice keeps the avocado from turning dark.

SERVES 8 | ¼ cup per serving

In a food processor or blender, process all the ingredients until smooth. Cover and refrigerate for at least 2 hours before serving.

10 ounces frozen shelled edamame (green soybeans), thawed

¾ cup cold water

½ medium avocado, chopped

¼ cup thinly sliced green onions

¼ cup snipped fresh cilantro

3 tablespoons fresh lime juice

1 medium garlic clove, minced

½ teaspoon ground cumin

¼ teaspoon salt

PER SERVING

calories 66	**cholesterol** 0 mg	**protein** 5 g	**dietary exchanges**
total fat 3.5 g	**sodium** 78 mg	**calcium** 24 mg	½ starch
saturated 0.5 g	**carbohydrates** 5 g	**potassium** 254 mg	½ lean meat
trans 0.0 g	fiber 3 g		
polyunsaturated 0.0 g	sugars 2 g		
monounsaturated 1.0 g			

HORSERADISH AND DILL SOUR CREAM DIP

Adding horseradish to sour cream and dill gives you a dip with zip!

SERVES 4 | ¼ cup per serving

In a small bowl, whisk together all the ingredients. Serve or cover and refrigerate until needed.

- ⅔ cup fat-free sour cream
- ¼ cup bottled white horseradish, drained
- ¼ cup fat-free milk
- 2 teaspoons dried dillweed, crumbled
- ⅛ teaspoon salt

PER SERVING

calories 49	**cholesterol** 7 mg	**protein** 3 g	**dietary exchanges**
total fat 0.0 g	**sodium** 129 mg	**calcium** 112 mg	½ other carbohydrate
saturated 0.0 g	**carbohydrates** 8 g	**potassium** 147 mg	
trans 0.0 g	fiber 0 g		
polyunsaturated 0.0 g	sugars 4 g		
monounsaturated 0.0 g			

WALDORF DIP

For a double dose of spice, serve this "scent-sational" dip with crisp gingersnaps. The combination is perfect as a slightly sweet appetizer or a bite of quick dessert.

SERVES 8 | ¼ cup per serving

In a medium bowl, stir together all the ingredients. Serve at room temperature or cover and refrigerate for up to three days. Stir gently just before serving if the mixture has become slightly watery.

COOK'S TIP ON DRY-ROASTING SEEDS, NUTS, OR WHOLE DRIED SPICES To dry-roast seeds, nuts, or dried spices, put them in a single layer in a small skillet. Cook over medium heat for about 4 minutes, or until the seeds darken and begin to pop, the nuts begin to brown, or the spices become very fragrant, stirring frequently. Remove them from the skillet so they don't burn.

8 ounces fat-free plain yogurt

1 medium apple, such as Granny Smith, Gala, or Fuji, peeled and finely chopped

1 medium rib of celery, finely chopped

¼ cup chopped walnuts, dry-roasted

1 tablespoon honey

1 teaspoon grated lemon zest

1 tablespoon fresh lemon juice

¼ teaspoon ground cinnamon

⅛ teaspoon ground nutmeg

PER SERVING

calories 58	**cholesterol** 1 mg	**protein** 2 g	**dietary exchanges**
total fat 2.5 g	**sodium** 26 mg	**calcium** 64 mg	½ other carbohydrate
saturated 0.5 g	**carbohydrates** 7 g	**potassium** 121 mg	½ fat
trans 0.0 g	fiber 1 g		
polyunsaturated 1.5 g	sugars 6 g		
monounsaturated 0.5 g			

HOT AND SMOKY CHIPOTLE-GARLIC DIP

This spicy mixture is delicious on cucumber rounds or unsalted baked corn tortillas.

SERVES 4 | ¼ cup per serving

In a food processor or blender, process all the ingredients except the cilantro until smooth. Transfer to a serving bowl. Garnish with the cilantro.

⅔ cup fat-free sour cream

3 tablespoons light mayonnaise

2 tablespoons fresh lemon juice

1 chipotle pepper canned in adobo sauce

1 medium garlic clove, minced

Sprigs of fresh cilantro (optional)

COOK'S TIP ON CHIPOTLE PEPPERS Chipotle peppers are dried jalapeños that are smoked to provide a unique heat. These flavorful chiles often are canned in adobo sauce, also known as adobo paste, a moderately spicy mixture of chiles, vinegar, garlic, and herbs. Dried chipotles also are sold in packages. To rehydrate them, put the desired number of chiles in a bowl of boiling water. Let stand for 20 minutes. Drain and use as directed above. You may want to keep the soaking water to spice up soup or beans.

PER SERVING

calories 73
total fat 3.0 g
  saturated 0.0 g
  trans 0.0 g
  polyunsaturated 2.0 g
  monounsaturated 0.5 g

cholesterol 10 mg
sodium 178 mg
carbohydrates 9 g
  fiber 0 g
  sugars 3 g

protein 3 g
calcium 82 mg
potassium 113 mg

dietary exchanges
  ½ other carbohydrate
  ½ fat

SPINACH-ARTICHOKE HUMMUS

Creamy texture, pretty green color, and assertive taste—this dip has it all!

SERVES 8 | ¼ cup per serving

In a food processor or blender, process all the ingredients until the desired consistency. Serve at room temperature or cover and refrigerate until needed.

COOK'S TIP ON TAHINI Tahini is a thick paste made from ground sesame seeds. Add small amounts to enhance salad dressings, marinades, soups, stuffings, and other dips and spreads. Look for tahini in the condiment or ethnic sections in the grocery store.

2 ounces spinach (about 2 cups)

1 cup canned no-salt-added chickpeas, rinsed and drained

4 medium canned artichoke hearts, rinsed, squeezed dry, and quartered

¼ cup Chicken Broth (page 50) or commercial fat-free, low-sodium chicken broth

2 tablespoons shredded or grated Parmesan cheese

½ teaspoon grated lemon zest

2 tablespoons fresh lemon juice

2 tablespoons tahini

1 to 2 medium garlic cloves, minced

¼ teaspoon pepper

PER SERVING

calories 101	cholesterol 1 mg	protein 5 g	dietary exchanges
total fat 3.5 g	sodium 89 mg	calcium 40 mg	1 starch
saturated 0.5 g	carbohydrates 13 g	potassium 188 mg	½ lean meat
trans 0.0 g	fiber 4 g		
polyunsaturated 1.5 g	sugars 2 g		
monounsaturated 1.5 g			

MUSHROOM-FILLED MINI PHYLLO SHELLS

Sautéed mixed mushrooms become delectable appetizers when you combine them with garlic, feta, and horseradish sauce, then use the filling in flaky mini phyllo shells.

SERVES 5 | 3 mini shells per serving

In a large nonstick skillet, heat the oil over medium-high heat, swirling to coat the bottom. Add the mushrooms, garlic, and brandy, stirring to combine. Cook for 5 to 6 minutes, or until the mushrooms are soft, stirring frequently. Increase the heat to high and cook for 1 to 2 minutes, or until the liquid has evaporated, stirring frequently.

Stir in the parsley and pepper. Remove from the heat.

Just before serving, spoon ¼ teaspoon feta into each phyllo shell. Top each with 1 heaping teaspoon mushroom mixture, then with ⅛ teaspoon horseradish sauce. Serve immediately.

1 teaspoon olive oil

4 ounces sliced button mushrooms

4 ounces sliced shiitake or brown (cremini) mushrooms, or a combination

3 medium garlic cloves, minced

3 tablespoons brandy or dry sherry (optional)

1 tablespoon minced fresh parsley

⅛ teaspoon pepper

1 tablespoon plus ¾ teaspoon crumbled fat-free feta cheese

15 frozen mini phyllo shells (1.90-ounce box), thawed

2 teaspoons (scant) bottled horseradish sauce (not bottled horseradish)

COOK'S TIP ON HORSERADISH SAUCE

Horseradish sauce, usually found in the condiment section of supermarkets, tastes much milder and has less heat than bottled horseradish. The sauce is similar to mayonnaise with a slight kick of horseradish but contains less fat and fewer calories.

PER SERVING

calories 98	cholesterol 2 mg	protein 2 g	dietary exchanges
total fat 4.5 g	sodium 82 mg	calcium 18 mg	½ starch
saturated 0.0 g	carbohydrates 8 g	potassium 157 mg	1 fat
trans 0.0 g	fiber 1 g		
polyunsaturated 1.0 g	sugars 1 g		
monounsaturated 1.5 g			

RED BELL PEPPER CROSTINI

By roasting bell peppers instead of using the bottled roasted variety, you will cut a lot of sodium from these crostini, or "little toasts." For an attractive presentation, arrange the hors d'oeuvres in a pinwheel design on a serving platter.

SERVES 8 | 2 crostini per serving

In a small mixing bowl, stir together the cream cheese, 1 tablespoon basil, milk, garlic, hot-pepper sauce, and salt. Using an electric mixer on medium speed, beat until smooth. Spread the mixture on the melba toast slices.

In another small bowl, stir together the bell peppers and vinegar. Sprinkle the bell pepper mixture and remaining 3 tablespoons basil over the melba toast slices.

2 ounces fat-free cream cheese

1 tablespoon chopped fresh basil or 1 teaspoon dried, crumbled, and 3 tablespoons chopped fresh basil or parsley, divided use

1 tablespoon fat-free milk

1 medium garlic clove, minced

¼ teaspoon red hot-pepper sauce

⅛ teaspoon salt

16 slices melba toast (lowest sodium available)

½ cup roasted red bell peppers, chopped

2 tablespoons cider vinegar

COOK'S TIP ON ROASTING BELL PEPPERS To "roast" bell peppers, preheat the broiler. Lightly spray a broiler pan and rack with cooking spray. Put the desired number of whole bell peppers on the rack; you'll need 2 medium red bell peppers for this recipe. Broil the peppers 3 to 4 inches from the heat, turning until the peppers are charred all over. Put the peppers in a bowl. Let stand, covered, for at least 5 minutes (it won't hurt the peppers to stand for as long as 20 minutes). Rinse with cold water and halve lengthwise. Using your fingers or a knife, peel off the skin (it's okay to leave small bits of char on the peppers). Discard the skin, stems, ribs, and seeds. Blot the peppers dry before chopping or slicing them.

PER SERVING

calories 50	**cholesterol** 1 mg	**protein** 2 g	**dietary exchanges**
total fat 0.5 g	**sodium** 98 mg	**calcium** 53 mg	½ starch
saturated 0.0 g	**carbohydrates** 9 g	**potassium** 62 mg	
trans 0.0 g	fiber 1 g		
polyunsaturated 0.0 g	sugars 0 g		
monounsaturated 0.0 g			

BAKED VEGGIE CHIPS

Lower in sodium than commercially baked chips, these crunchy snacks are very easy to make, especially if you have a mandolin or a food processor to slice the veggies quickly and uniformly.

SERVES 4 | ½ cup per serving

Preheat the oven to 375°F.

In a large bowl, gently stir together all the ingredients except the salt. Place the vegetable slices close together in a single layer on two large baking sheets.

Bake for 30 to 35 minutes, or until browned, checking closely during the last 10 minutes to keep the chips from burning and transferring them to a medium bowl as they become ready. They will crisp as they cool, about 5 minutes.

Sprinkle the chips with the salt, gently stirring to coat.

1 **small sweet potato,** cut crosswise into ¹⁄₁₆-inch slices

1 **small baking potato,** cut crosswise into ¹⁄₁₆-inch slices

1 **large parsnip, peeled** and cut crosswise into ¹⁄₁₆-inch slices

1 **large carrot, peeled** and cut crosswise into ¹⁄₁₆-inch slices

2 **teaspoons olive oil**

⅛ **teaspoon salt**

COOK'S TIP The chips will lose their crispness when stored, so they are best on the day they are made. If you keep the chips for another time, however, you can restore their crispness by putting them on a baking sheet and baking at 250°F for 8 to 10 minutes.

PER SERVING

calories 110	**cholesterol** 0 mg	**protein** 2 g	**dietary exchanges**
total fat 2.5 g	**sodium** 111 mg	**calcium** 32 mg	1½ starch
saturated 0.5 g	**carbohydrates** 21 g	**potassium** 464 mg	
trans 0.0 g	fiber 4 g		
polyunsaturated 0.5 g	sugars 4 g		
monounsaturated 1.5 g			

PARTY MIX

Get hooked on this crunchy, low-salt snack mix and use it to replace high-sodium potato chips.

SERVES 12 | ¼ cup per serving

Preheat the oven to 400°F.

In a large bowl, stir together the cereal squares, pretzels, bagel chips, and peanuts.

In a small bowl, whisk together the Worcestershire sauce, mustard, oil, garlic powder, cumin, and cayenne. Stir into the cereal mixture. Spread in a single layer on a rimmed baking sheet.

Bake for 4 minutes, stirring once halfway through. Transfer the baking sheet to a cooling rack.

Lightly spray the mixture with cooking spray. Sprinkle with the salt. Let cool on the cooling rack. The mixture will become crisp as it cools, about 10 minutes.

1¼ cups corn cereal squares (lowest sodium available)

¾ cup bite-size shredded wheat cereal squares (lowest sodium available)

½ cup thin unsalted pretzel sticks

2 low-sodium bagel chips, broken into ½-inch pieces (about ½ cup)

¼ cup unsalted peanuts

1½ tablespoons Worcestershire sauce (lowest sodium available)

1 tablespoon honey mustard (lowest sodium available)

2 teaspoons toasted sesame oil

½ teaspoon garlic powder

½ teaspoon ground cumin

⅛ teaspoon cayenne

Cooking spray

¼ teaspoon salt

PER SERVING

calories 69	**cholesterol** 0 mg	**protein** 2 g	**dietary exchanges**
total fat 2.5 g	**sodium** 121 mg	**calcium** 22 mg	½ starch
saturated 0.5 g	**carbohydrates** 10 g	**potassium** 55 mg	½ fat
trans 0.0 g	fiber 1 g		
polyunsaturated 1.0 g	sugars 1 g		
monounsaturated 1.0 g			

MELON-BERRY KEBABS

Attractive, fragrant, and so tasty, these kebabs are a great way to fit more servings of fruit into your diet.

SERVES 4 | 1 kebab per serving

In a small microwaveable bowl, microwave the lemon juice on 100 percent power (high) for 15 seconds, or until hot. Stir in the lemon zest, sugar, and gingerroot. Set aside to cool.

Stir the mint into the lemon juice mixture. Using the back of a spoon, mash the mint to release the flavor. Pour into a pie pan.

Add the melon and strawberries to the lemon juice mixture, gently stirring to coat.

Using 3 melon cubes and 2 strawberries per skewer, alternate the fruit as you thread it onto four 6-inch wooden skewers.

2 tablespoons fresh lemon juice

½ teaspoon grated lemon zest

1 tablespoon sugar

1½ teaspoons grated peeled gingerroot

2 tablespoons chopped fresh mint

12 1-inch watermelon or honeydew cubes

8 whole strawberries, hulled

COOK'S TIP You may want to add a whole mint leaf at the base of each kebab. The dark green leaves provide a nice color contrast and keep your fingers from touching the sticky fruit.

PER SERVING

calories 32	**cholesterol** 0 mg	**protein** 1 g	**dietary exchanges**
total fat 0.0 g	**sodium** 2 mg	**calcium** 14 mg	½ fruit
saturated 0.0 g	**carbohydrates** 8 g	**potassium** 82 mg	
trans 0.0 g	fiber 1 g		
polyunsaturated 0.0 g	sugars 6 g		
monounsaturated 0.0 g			

SOUPS

CHICKEN BROTH

With this big batch of broth, you'll have plenty to serve as a first course and to freeze for later use in a variety of recipes. Save the cooked chicken for Chicken Salad (page 91) or Chicken, Barley, and Spinach Casserole (page 160).

SERVES 12 | ¾ cup per serving

In a stockpot, stir together all the ingredients. Bring to a boil over high heat. Skim any foam off the top. Reduce the heat and simmer, covered, for 1 to 2 hours if not using the extra bones or 3 to 4 hours with the extra bones (to prevent cloudiness, don't let the broth return to a boil).

Remove the chicken and reserve for another use. Discard the bones. Strain the broth into an airtight container, discarding the vegetables, peppercorns, and bay leaf. Cover and refrigerate the broth for 1 to 2 hours, or until the fat hardens on the surface. Discard the hardened fat before reheating the broth.

3 pounds skinless chicken pieces with bones, all visible fat discarded

2 to 3 pounds chicken bones (optional)

3 quarts water

2 large carrots, chopped

2 medium ribs of celery, sliced

1 medium onion, chopped

5 or 6 whole peppercorns

1 medium dried bay leaf

1 teaspoon dried thyme, crumbled

¼ teaspoon pepper

COOK'S TIP ON FREEZING BROTH Freeze broth in airtight containers to use by itself or as the base for other soups. Freeze small amounts of leftover broth in ice cube trays for future use as an ideal low-sodium seasoning. Put 1 tablespoon of broth in each compartment of the tray, then freeze. Remove the broth cubes from the tray and store them in an airtight plastic freezer bag so you'll have a tablespoon at a time whenever you need it. For some recipes, such as soups that use just a small amount of broth, you can toss in the still-frozen cubes. For dishes such as casseroles, first thaw the cubes in the microwave or for several hours in the refrigerator.

COOK'S TIP ON LOW-SODIUM BROTH This broth, Beef Broth (page 52), and Vegetable Broth (page 53) are much lower in sodium than most commercially available low-sodium broths, so it's a good idea to have plenty of these homemade broths on hand.

PER SERVING

calories 8	**cholesterol** 0 mg	**protein** 2 g	**dietary exchanges**
total fat 0.0 g	**sodium** 19 mg	**calcium** 4 mg	free
saturated 0.0 g	**carbohydrates** 0 g	**potassium** 75 mg	
trans 0.0 g	fiber 0 g		
polyunsaturated 0.0 g	sugars 0 g		
monounsaturated 0.0 g			

BEEF BROTH

Beef broth is good "as is" and for adding flavor to many dishes. Roasting the bones adds both flavor and color to the broth. Keep some broth in the freezer so you'll have it whenever you need it (see Cook's Tip on Freezing Broth, page 51).

SERVES 12 | ¾ cup per serving

Preheat the oven to 400°F. Lightly spray a roasting pan with cooking spray.

Put the bones in the pan.

Roast for 25 to 30 minutes, turning once halfway through. Using tongs, transfer the bones to a stockpot.

Add the remaining ingredients to the pot. Bring to a boil over high heat. Skim any foam off the top. Reduce the heat and simmer, covered, for 4 to 6 hours (to prevent cloudiness, don't let the broth return to a boil). Strain the broth into an airtight container, discarding the solids. Cover and refrigerate the broth for 1 to 2 hours, or until the fat hardens on the surface. Discard the hardened fat before reheating the broth.

Cooking spray

4 pounds beef or veal bones (preferably shank or knuckle bones)

3 quarts water

1 medium onion, coarsely chopped

8 sprigs of fresh parsley

1 teaspoon dried thyme, crumbled

5 or 6 whole peppercorns

2 whole cloves

1 medium dried bay leaf

PER SERVING

calories 8	cholesterol 0 mg	protein 2 g	dietary exchanges
total fat 0.0 g	sodium 23 mg	calcium 8 mg	free
saturated 0.0 g	carbohydrates 0 g	potassium 75 mg	
trans 0.0 g	fiber 0 g		
polyunsaturated 0.0 g	sugars 0 g		
monounsaturated 0.0 g			

VEGETABLE BROTH

For a flavor change, replace beef or chicken broth with this tasty, so-easy-to-make broth. If you have extra broth, see the Cook's Tip on Freezing Broth (page 51).

SERVES 8 | ¾ cup per serving

In a stockpot, stir together all the ingredients. Bring to a simmer over medium-high heat (to prevent cloudiness, don't let the broth reach a boil). Reduce the heat and simmer, covered, for 1 hour. Strain the broth into an airtight container, discarding the trimmings. Cover and refrigerate so the flavors blend. Reheat before serving.

4 cups vegetable trimmings, such as carrots, celery, tomatoes, onions, spinach, and leeks
6 cups water
⅛ to ¼ teaspoon pepper

COOK'S TIP Keep a large airtight plastic bag in the freezer and use it for collecting vegetable peels and trimmed ends. When it's time to make this broth, your veggies will be waiting.

PER SERVING

calories 6	cholesterol 0 mg	protein 1 g	dietary exchanges
total fat 0.0 g	sodium 18 mg	calcium 3 mg	free
saturated 0.0 g	carbohydrates 1 g	potassium 20 mg	
trans 0.0 g	fiber 0 g		
polyunsaturated 0.0 g	sugars 0 g		
monounsaturated 0.0 g			

BLACK BEAN SOUP

Pair this smooth, cumin-rich soup with unsalted baked corn tortilla strips and a deep green salad for a simple, hearty meal.

SERVES 10 | 1 cup per serving

In a stockpot, heat the oil over medium-high heat, swirling to coat the bottom. Cook the onions for 3 minutes, or until soft, stirring frequently. Reduce the heat to medium.

Stir in the celery and garlic. Cook for 4 minutes, stirring frequently.

Stir in the beans and reserved liquid. Stir in the remaining ingredients except the sour cream. Increase the heat to high and bring to a boil. Reduce the heat and simmer, covered, for 25 minutes. Remove from the heat.

In a food processor or blender, process the soup in batches until smooth. Serve with dollops of sour cream.

1 tablespoon olive oil

3 to 4 medium onions, chopped

3 medium ribs of celery, diced

5 large garlic cloves, chopped

3 15.5-ounce cans no-salt-added black beans, 1 cup liquid reserved (add water if needed), beans rinsed and drained

4 cups Chicken Broth (page 50) or commercial fat-free, low-sodium chicken broth

1 28-ounce can no-salt-added stewed tomatoes, undrained

1 tablespoon ground cumin

1½ teaspoons dried cilantro, crumbled

⅛ to ¼ teaspoon cayenne

½ cup fat-free sour cream, lightly beaten with a fork until smooth

PER SERVING

calories 146
total fat 1.5 g
  saturated 0.0 g
  trans 0.0 g
  polyunsaturated 0.0 g
  monounsaturated 1.0 g

cholesterol 2 mg
sodium 43 mg
carbohydrates 30 g
  fiber 9 g
  sugars 9 g

protein 8 g
calcium 122 mg
potassium 658 mg

dietary exchanges
1½ starch
2 vegetable
½ very lean meat

CREAMY CARROT SOUP

Beautiful in color, this soup is creamy without using dairy products. The crunchy pumpkin seeds provide a nice texture contrast. Serve the soup hot in the winter and chilled in the summer.

SERVES 5 | 1 cup per serving

In a stockpot, heat the oil over medium heat, swirling to coat the bottom. Cook the onions for 2 to 3 minutes, or until soft, stirring occasionally.

Stir in the carrots. Cook for 1 to 2 minutes, stirring occasionally.

Pour in the broth. Increase the heat to high and bring to a boil. Reduce the heat and simmer for 30 minutes, or until the carrots are tender. Remove from the heat. Stir in the cayenne.

In a food processor or blender, process the soup in batches until smooth. To serve hot, sprinkle with the pumpkin seeds and green onions. To serve chilled, transfer the soup to an airtight container and refrigerate until needed. Sprinkle with the pumpkin seeds and green onions at serving time.

1 tablespoon olive oil

2 cups thinly sliced sweet onions, such as Vidalia, Maui, or Oso Sweet

3 cups thickly sliced carrots

4 cups Chicken Broth (page 50) or commercial fat-free, low-sodium chicken broth

Dash of cayenne

1 tablespoon unsalted shelled pumpkin seeds

Chopped green onions (green part only; optional)

PER SERVING

calories 90	**cholesterol** 0 mg	**protein** 3 g	**dietary exchanges**
total fat 3.5 g	**sodium** 73 mg	**calcium** 40 mg	2 vegetable
saturated 0.5 g	**carbohydrates** 12 g	**potassium** 395 mg	1 fat
trans 0.0 g	fiber 3 g		
polyunsaturated 0.5 g	sugars 5 g		
monounsaturated 2.0 g			

CORN AND GREEN CHILE SOUP

Ready in no time, this chunky and spicy soup requires very little cleanup.

SERVES 4 | heaping ¾ cup per serving

In a medium saucepan, stir together the corn, milk, green chiles, cumin, pepper, and cayenne. Bring just to a simmer over medium heat, stirring frequently. Remove from the heat.

Stir in the bell pepper, green onions, and margarine. Serve sprinkled with the Cheddar.

16 ounces frozen whole-kernel corn, thawed

12 ounces fat-free evaporated milk

2 ounces chopped green chiles, drained

¼ to ½ teaspoon ground cumin

¼ teaspoon pepper

⅛ teaspoon cayenne (optional)

½ medium red bell pepper, finely chopped (optional)

3 medium green onions, finely chopped

2 teaspoons light tub margarine

¼ cup shredded fat-free sharp Cheddar cheese

COOK'S TIP ON THAWING FROZEN VEGETABLES To thaw frozen vegetables quickly, put them in a colander and run them under cold water until thawed. Shake off the excess water and drain well.

PER SERVING

calories 208	**cholesterol** 5 mg	**protein** 13 g	**dietary exchanges**
total fat 2.0 g	**sodium** 256 mg	**calcium** 358 mg	1½ starch
saturated 0.5 g	**carbohydrates** 38 g	**potassium** 658 mg	1 fat-free milk
trans 0.0 g	fiber 4 g		
polyunsaturated 0.5 g	sugars 15 g		
monounsaturated 0.5 g			

THAI SWEET-POTATO SOUP

A touch of spicy curry paste makes this sweet-potato soup sing. It is an obvious choice to serve with Asian food, but don't overlook it for other meals as well. Try the soup with roasted turkey for Thanksgiving, serve it tonight with Pork Chops with Herb Rub (page 196), or warm up a fall picnic by sharing some of it from an insulated container.

SERVES 4 | 1 cup per serving

In a large saucepan, heat the oil over medium-high heat, swirling to coat the bottom. Cook the onion for 3 minutes, or until soft, stirring frequently.

Stir in the garlic. Cook for 1 minute, stirring constantly.

Stir in the broth and sweet potatoes. Bring to a simmer. Reduce the heat and simmer, covered, for 15 to 20 minutes, or until the sweet potatoes are very tender. Stir in the curry paste.

In a food processor or blender, process the soup in batches until smooth. Stir in the lime juice.

- 2 teaspoons canola or corn oil
- 1 small onion, chopped
- 1 medium garlic clove, chopped
- 3 cups Vegetable Broth (page 53) or commercial low-sodium vegetable broth
- ¾ pound sweet potatoes, peeled and chopped (about 2½ cups)
- ½ teaspoon Thai red curry paste
- 1 tablespoon fresh lime juice

PER SERVING

calories 114	**cholesterol** 0 mg	**protein** 3 g	**dietary exchanges**
total fat 2.5 g	**sodium** 77 mg	**calcium** 38 mg	1½ starch
saturated 0.0 g	**carbohydrates** 21 g	**potassium** 360 mg	
trans 0.0 g	fiber 3 g		
polyunsaturated 0.5 g	sugars 5 g		
monounsaturated 1.5 g			

FRESH BASIL, SPINACH, AND TOMATO SOUP

Just a few minutes of standing time brings out the delectable flavor of the fresh basil in this easy-to-prepare soup.

SERVES 4 | ¾ cup per serving

In a medium saucepan, stir together the broth, oregano, garlic, tarragon, and red pepper flakes. Bring to a boil over high heat. Reduce the heat and simmer for 5 minutes. Remove from the heat.

Stir in the remaining ingredients except the lemon slices. Let stand, covered, for 5 minutes so the flavors blend. Serve garnished with the lemon slices. For peak flavor, serve immediately after the standing time.

- 2 cups Chicken Broth (page 50) or commercial fat-free, low-sodium chicken broth
- 1 teaspoon dried oregano, crumbled
- 1 medium garlic clove, minced
- ¼ teaspoon dried tarragon, crumbled
- ⅛ teaspoon crushed red pepper flakes (optional)
- 4 small tomatoes, diced
- 2 ounces spinach (about 2 cups), coarsely chopped
- 2 medium green onions, finely chopped
- ¼ cup chopped fresh basil (about ⅓ ounce)
- ½ teaspoon olive oil (extra virgin preferred)
- ⅛ teaspoon salt
- 4 lemon slices (optional)

PER SERVING

calories 38	**cholesterol** 0 mg	**protein** 2 g	**dietary exchanges**
total fat 1.0 g	**sodium** 104 mg	**calcium** 37 mg	1 vegetable
saturated 0.0 g	**carbohydrates** 6 g	**potassium** 399 mg	
trans 0.0 g	fiber 2 g		
polyunsaturated 0.0 g	sugars 3 g		
monounsaturated 0.5 g			

GAZPACHO

When the dog days of summer arrive, turn to this no-cook chilled soup. It is low in sodium and calories, contains no fat, and is quite refreshing.

SERVES 12 | ½ cup per serving

Finely chop the cucumbers, tomato, bell pepper, zucchini, onion, and green onions. Put in a large bowl.

Stir in the remaining ingredients except the lemon wedges. Cover and refrigerate for at least 2 hours. Serve with the lemon wedges on the side.

2 medium cucumbers

1 medium tomato

1 small green bell pepper

1 small zucchini

½ medium onion

3 or 4 medium green onions

4 cups low-sodium mixed-vegetable juice

¼ cup snipped fresh parsley or 1 tablespoon plus 1 teaspoon dried, crumbled

1 tablespoon fresh lemon juice (optional)

2 medium garlic cloves, minced

1 teaspoon Worcestershire sauce (lowest sodium available)

½ to 1 teaspoon pepper

1½ medium lemons, cut into 12 wedges total (optional)

PER SERVING

calories 33	**cholesterol** 0 mg	**protein** 2 g	**dietary exchanges**
total fat 0.0 g	**sodium** 52 mg	**calcium** 25 mg	1 vegetable
saturated 0.0 g	**carbohydrates** 7 g	**potassium** 444 mg	
trans 0.0 g	fiber 2 g		
polyunsaturated 0.0 g	sugars 5 g		
monounsaturated 0.0 g			

SOUP TO GO

Here's how to have a quick cup of soup that won't eat up your sodium limit for the day. Keep this mixture on hand at work for an easy lunch or take it on a camping trip—in fact, you can use it wherever boiling water is available.

SERVES 1 | 1 cup per serving

In a small airtight plastic bag or container, stir together all the ingredients for the chicken or beef soup mix.

To prepare the soup, put the dry mixture in a soup bowl. Pour in the boiling water. Stir. Let stand for 1 to 2 minutes, or until the rice is tender.

CHICKEN SOUP TO GO MIX

- ¼ cup uncooked instant brown rice or 2 tablespoons uncooked whole-wheat couscous
- ¼ cup no-salt-added mixed dried vegetables, such as carrots, tomatoes, green peas, and corn
- 1½ teaspoons very low sodium chicken bouillon granules
- ½ teaspoon dried parsley, crumbled
- ½ teaspoon dried minced onion
- ⅛ teaspoon dried thyme, crumbled
- ⅛ teaspoon pepper

OR

BEEF SOUP TO GO MIX

- ¼ cup uncooked instant brown rice or 2 tablespoons uncooked whole-wheat couscous
- ¼ cup no-salt-added mixed dried vegetables, such as carrots, tomatoes, green peas, and corn
- 1½ teaspoons very low sodium beef bouillon granules
- 1 teaspoon dried shallots
- ½ teaspoon dried parsley, crumbled
- ⅛ teaspoon dried marjoram, crumbled
- ⅛ teaspoon pepper

- 1 cup boiling water

COOK'S TIP Experiment with different dried vegetables (often located with the fresh produce in the grocery store) and no-salt-added herb or seasoning combinations. Keep a small bottle of toasted sesame oil handy and pour a few drops into the chicken soup for an Asian flavor (similar to that of egg drop soup).

COOK'S TIP If you begin with new jars of herbs and bouillon granules, these soup mixtures will keep in an airtight container for up to a year. Be sure to keep them in a closed cabinet away from the light.

PER SERVING
CHICKEN SOUP

calories 184	**cholesterol** 0 mg	**protein** 5 g	**dietary exchanges**
total fat 1.5 g	**sodium** 46 mg	**calcium** 43 mg	1½ starch
saturated 0.0 g	**carbohydrates** 38 g	**potassium** 1,196 mg	3 vegetable
trans 0.0 g	fiber 3 g		
polyunsaturated 0.5 g	sugars 0 g		
monounsaturated 0.5 g			

PER SERVING
BEEF SOUP

calories 183	**cholesterol** 0 mg	**protein** 5 g	**dietary exchanges**
total fat 1.5 g	**sodium** 53 mg	**calcium** 42 mg	1½ starch
saturated 0.0 g	**carbohydrates** 37 g	**potassium** 1,146 mg	3 vegetable
trans 0.0 g	fiber 3 g		
polyunsaturated 0.5 g	sugars 2 g		
monounsaturated 0.5 g			

MINESTRONE

Enjoy a bowl of this soup for a light lunch, or pair it with a dark green or spinach salad or Balsamic-Marinated Vegetables (page 78) for a heartier meal.

SERVES 10 | 1 cup per serving

Lightly spray a stockpot with olive oil spray. Add the oil, swirling to coat the bottom. Cook the onion, carrot, celery, and garlic over medium heat for 3 to 4 minutes, or until the onion is soft, stirring occasionally.

Stir in the remaining ingredients except the Parmesan. Bring to a simmer. Simmer, covered, for 5 minutes, or until heated through. Serve sprinkled with the Parmesan.

Olive oil spray

1½ teaspoons olive oil

1 small onion, chopped

1 medium carrot, thinly sliced

1 medium rib of celery, diced

1 to 2 medium garlic cloves, minced

6 cups Chicken Broth (page 50) or commercial fat-free, low-sodium chicken broth

1 cup canned no-salt-added diced tomatoes, drained

1 cup cooked whole-grain macaroni (cooked without salt)

1 cup canned no-salt-added white beans, such as cannellini beans, rinsed and drained

½ teaspoon pepper

¼ cup shredded or grated Parmesan cheese

PER SERVING

calories 73	**cholesterol** 1 mg	**protein** 5 g	**dietary exchanges**
total fat 1.5 g	**sodium** 60 mg	**calcium** 53 mg	½ starch
saturated 0.5 g	**carbohydrates** 11 g	**potassium** 268 mg	½ very lean meat
trans 0.0 g	fiber 2 g		
polyunsaturated 0.0 g	sugars 3 g		
monounsaturated 0.5 g			

NEW ENGLAND FISH CHOWDER with Thyme

This creamy chowder boasts chunks of potato and your favorite mild white fish. For a little crunch, top it with crumbled no-salt-added pretzels.

SERVES 6 | 1 cup per serving

In a large saucepan, heat the oil over medium-high heat, swirling to coat the bottom. Cook the onion for 3 minutes, or until soft, stirring frequently.

Stir in the fish stock, potatoes, thyme, and pepper. Bring to a simmer. Reduce the heat and simmer, covered, for 20 to 25 minutes, or until the potatoes are tender.

In a small bowl, whisk together the milk and flour. Whisk into the stock mixture. Increase the heat to medium high and cook for about 5 minutes, or until the mixture thickens, stirring occasionally. Reduce the heat to medium.

Stir in the fish. Cook for 6 to 7 minutes, or until the fish flakes easily when tested with a fork, stirring occasionally.

2 teaspoons canola or corn oil

1 medium onion, chopped

3 cups low-sodium fish stock, Chicken Broth (page 50), or commercial fat-free, low-sodium chicken broth

2 medium potatoes, peeled and cut into ½-inch cubes (about 1½ cups)

¾ teaspoon dried thyme, crumbled

⅛ teaspoon pepper (white preferred)

1 cup fat-free evaporated milk

¼ cup all-purpose flour

1 pound firm mild white fish fillets, such as haddock or cod, rinsed and patted dry, cut into ½-inch cubes

PER SERVING

calories 181	**cholesterol** 45 mg	**protein** 20 g	**dietary exchanges**
total fat 2.0 g	**sodium** 114 mg	**calcium** 167 mg	1 starch
saturated 0.5 g	**carbohydrates** 20 g	**potassium** 672 mg	½ fat-free milk
trans 0.0 g	fiber 1 g		2 very lean meat
polyunsaturated 0.5 g	sugars 7 g		
monounsaturated 1.0 g			

TURKEY VEGETABLE SOUP

Here's a good way to use up some of that leftover holiday turkey!

SERVES 6 | 1½ cups per serving

Lightly spray a stockpot with cooking spray. Put the oil in the pot, swirling to coat the bottom. Cook the onion and celery over medium-high heat for 3 minutes, or until the onion is soft, stirring frequently.

Stir in the remaining ingredients. Increase the heat to high and bring to a simmer. Reduce the heat and simmer, covered, for 20 minutes.

Cooking spray

1 teaspoon canola or corn oil

1 medium onion, chopped

½ medium rib of celery, diced

6 cups Chicken Broth (page 50) or commercial fat-free, low-sodium chicken broth

1 cup canned no-salt-added diced tomatoes, drained

1 cup chopped cooked turkey breast, cooked without salt, all visible fat and skin discarded

½ cup frozen green peas

½ cup frozen whole-kernel corn

½ teaspoon pepper

¼ teaspoon red hot-pepper sauce

PER SERVING

calories 84	**cholesterol** 20 mg	**protein** 11 g	**dietary exchanges**
total fat 1.5 g	**sodium** 59 mg	**calcium** 32 mg	½ starch
saturated 0.0 g	**carbohydrates** 8 g	**potassium** 340 mg	1 very lean meat
trans 0.0 g	fiber 2 g		
polyunsaturated 0.5 g	sugars 3 g		
monounsaturated 0.5 g			

CHICKEN, VEGETABLE, AND BARLEY SOUP

A garden of vegetables teams up with barley and lean chicken to make this "souper" nutritious. The cooking water from the chicken serves as a flavorful low-salt base for the soup.

SERVES 4 | 1½ cups per serving

In a small saucepan, combine 1 cup water and the barley. Bring to a boil over high heat. Reduce the heat and simmer, covered, for 15 to 20 minutes, or until the barley is tender. Drain and rinse in a colander. Set aside.

Meanwhile, in a medium saucepan, stir together the chicken, onion, garlic, salt, pepper, and remaining 2 cups water. Bring to a boil over high heat. Reduce the heat and simmer, covered, for 12 to 15 minutes, or until the chicken is no longer pink in the center. Transfer the chicken to a cutting board, leaving the remaining soup in the pan. Set the chicken aside.

Stir the tomatoes with liquid, zucchini, and yellow squash into the soup. Simmer, covered, for 5 minutes, or until the zucchini and yellow squash are tender. Meanwhile, dice the chicken. When the squashes are tender, stir the chicken, barley, and spinach into the soup. Cook for 2 minutes, or just until the spinach wilts. Remove from the heat. Stir in the lemon juice.

1 cup water and 2 cups water, divided use

¼ cup uncooked pearl barley

1 pound boneless, skinless chicken breasts, all visible fat discarded

½ cup chopped onion

2 medium garlic cloves, minced

¼ teaspoon salt

¼ teaspoon pepper

1 14.5-ounce can no-salt-added diced tomatoes, undrained

1 small zucchini, chopped

1 small yellow summer squash, chopped

2 ounces spinach (about 2 cups), coarsely chopped

3 tablespoons fresh lemon juice

PER SERVING

calories 219	**cholesterol** 66 mg	**protein** 30 g	**dietary exchanges**
total fat 1.5 g	**sodium** 253 mg	**calcium** 69 mg	½ starch
saturated 0.5 g	**carbohydrates** 20 g	**potassium** 804 mg	2 vegetable
trans 0.0 g	fiber 4 g		3 very lean meat
polyunsaturated 0.5 g	sugars 6 g		
monounsaturated 0.5 g			

LEMON-DILL CHICKEN AND RICE SOUP with Carrots and Asparagus

Fresh asparagus and dill turn this soup into a flavorful celebration of spring.

SERVES 4 | 1½ heaping cups per serving

In a small saucepan, combine the rice and ½ cup water. Cook using the package directions. Remove from the heat. Set aside.

Meanwhile, in a medium saucepan, stir together 2 cups water, the chicken, garlic, salt, and pepper. Bring to a boil over high heat. Reduce the heat and simmer, covered, for 12 to 15 minutes, or until the chicken is no longer pink in the center. Transfer the chicken to a cutting board, leaving the remaining soup in the pan. Set the chicken aside.

Pour the final 2 cups water into the pan. Increase the heat to high and bring to a boil. Add the carrots. Reduce the heat and simmer, covered, for 5 minutes, or until the carrots are tender.

¼ cup uncooked instant brown rice

½ cup water, 2 cups water, and 2 cups water, divided use

1 pound boneless, skinless chicken breasts, all visible fat discarded

2 medium garlic cloves, minced

¼ teaspoon salt

⅛ teaspoon pepper

2 large carrots, halved lengthwise and sliced crosswise

8 ounces asparagus, trimmed and cut crosswise into 1-inch pieces

2 tablespoons coarsely snipped fresh dillweed

2 tablespoons fresh lemon juice

1 medium green onion, thinly sliced

Meanwhile, dice the chicken. When the carrots are ready, add the chicken and asparagus to the soup. Return to a simmer. Reduce the heat and simmer, covered, for 3 minutes, or until the asparagus is crisp-tender. Remove from the heat.

Stir in the rice, dillweed, lemon juice, and green onion.

COOK'S TIP ON TRIMMING ASPARAGUS Asparagus has a natural bending point where the tough part of the stem begins. To trim asparagus, hold the spears at the top and the bottom, bend them, and snap at the bending point. Save the tough parts for use in making Vegetable Broth (page 53) or discard them.

PER SERVING

calories 179	**cholesterol** 66 mg	**protein** 28 g	**dietary exchanges**
total fat 2.0 g	**sodium** 256 mg	**calcium** 50 mg	½ starch
saturated 0.5 g	**carbohydrates** 12 g	**potassium** 562 mg	1 vegetable
trans 0.0 g	fiber 3 g		3 very lean meat
polyunsaturated 0.5 g	sugars 3 g		
monounsaturated 0.5 g			

VEGETABLE BEEF SOUP

Making this soup with roast beef you've saved from another meal (maybe Easy Roast Beef, page 170) cuts down on both prep time and cooking time. Even people who think they don't like leftovers will enjoy this soup, which gets lots of flavor from fresh produce.

SERVES 6 | 1 cup per serving

Lightly spray a Dutch oven with cooking spray. Cook the onion, celery, carrot, oregano, garlic, and thyme over medium heat for 4 minutes, or until the onion is soft, stirring occasionally.

Stir in the remaining ingredients. Bring to a simmer. Reduce the heat and simmer, covered, for 30 minutes, or until the vegetables are tender.

COOK'S TIP ON THICKENING SOUP To thicken and enrich most kinds of soup, either add some vegetables if none are called for or use more vegetables than the recipe specifies. Once they've cooked, transfer some or all of the vegetables to a food processor or blender and process until smooth, adding a little liquid if needed. Stir the processed vegetables back into the soup.

Cooking spray
- 1 medium onion, chopped
- 1 medium rib of celery, diced
- 1 medium carrot, sliced
- 1½ teaspoons chopped fresh oregano or ½ teaspoon dried, crumbled
- 2 medium garlic cloves, minced
- ½ teaspoon dried thyme, crumbled
- 4 cups Beef Broth (page 52) or commercial fat-free, no-salt-added beef broth
- 1 cup chopped cooked lean roast beef, cooked without salt, all visible fat discarded
- 1 cup cut fresh or frozen green beans
- 1 medium tomato, chopped

Pepper to taste

PER SERVING

calories 70	**cholesterol** 13 mg	**protein** 9 g	**dietary exchanges**
total fat 1.0 g	**sodium** 46 mg	**calcium** 35 mg	1 vegetable
saturated 0.5 g	**carbohydrates** 6 g	**potassium** 304 mg	1 very lean meat
trans 0.0 g	fiber 2 g		
polyunsaturated 0.0 g	sugars 3 g		
monounsaturated 0.5 g			

CURRIED SPLIT PEA SOUP

Curry powder and ground cumin add an unexpected flair to traditional split pea soup.

SERVES 6 | 1 cup per serving

In a Dutch oven, stir together all the ingredients except the salt. Bring to a boil over high heat. Reduce the heat and simmer, covered, for 1 hour to 1 hour 30 minutes, or until the peas are tender (no stirring needed).

Whisk in the salt. Whisk vigorously (but carefully, so you don't burn yourself) to slightly mash the peas, thickening the soup to the desired consistency.

6 cups Chicken Broth (page 50), Beef Broth (page 52), Vegetable Broth (page 53), or commercial low-sodium broth

1 cup dried split peas, sorted for stones and shriveled peas, rinsed, and drained

2 medium carrots, chopped

1 large onion, chopped

1½ teaspoons sugar

1½ teaspoons curry powder

1 teaspoon ground cumin

⅛ teaspoon garlic powder

⅛ teaspoon cayenne

¾ teaspoon salt

PER SERVING

calories 153
total fat 0.5 g
  saturated 0.0 g
  trans 0.0 g
  polyunsaturated 0.0 g
  monounsaturated 0.0 g

cholesterol 0 mg
sodium 339 mg
carbohydrates 27 g
  fiber 10 g
  sugars 7 g

protein 11 g
calcium 46 mg
potassium 568 mg

dietary exchanges
1½ starch
1 vegetable
½ very lean meat

LIMA BEAN SOUP
with Ham Bits and Crisp Sage

Fresh sage garnish, lightly crisped on the stovetop, updates humble lima bean soup and gives it restaurant-like flair.

SERVES 6 | 1½ cups per serving

Put the beans in a Dutch oven. Cover with 2 inches of water (this is not the 4 cups water). Bring to a boil over medium-high heat. Boil for 2 minutes. Remove from the heat. Let stand, covered, for 1 hour. Drain in a colander. Return the beans to the pot.

Stir in 4 cups water, the onion, ham, garlic, and bay leaves. Bring to a boil over medium-high heat. Reduce the heat and simmer, covered, for 1 hour, stirring occasionally. Discard the bay leaves.

Stir in the carrots and salt. Increase the heat to medium high and return to a simmer. Simmer, uncovered, for 20 minutes, or until the beans and carrots are tender.

For a creamier texture, transfer about 2 cups soup to a medium bowl. Mash the soup with a potato masher. Stir the mashed soup into the soup in the pot. For a smoother soup, in a food processor or blender, process all the soup in batches (without mashing any beans first) until the desired consistency.

16 ounces dried baby lima beans (about 2½ cups), sorted for stones and shriveled beans, rinsed, and drained

4 cups water

1 large onion, chopped

½ cup diced lower-sodium, low-fat ham, all visible fat discarded

4 medium garlic cloves, minced

2 medium dried bay leaves

5 medium carrots, shredded (about 2½ cups)

¼ teaspoon salt

1 teaspoon olive oil

12 fresh sage leaves

Meanwhile, in a small nonstick skillet, heat the oil over medium heat, swirling to coat the bottom. Cook the sage for 1 to 2 minutes, or until crisp, stirring frequently. Transfer the sage to paper towels and drain. Crumble and set aside. Use to garnish the soup.

COOK'S TIP Most individuals need about 4,700 milligrams of potassium daily to help keep blood pressure levels at a healthy level. A serving of this soup provides almost one-fourth of that amount, primarily because of the lima beans.

COOK'S TIP ON HAM Like other processed meats, ham usually is extremely high in sodium. When you shop, be sure to read product labels and select ham with the lowest amounts of sodium, saturated fat, and cholesterol. It doesn't take much ham to provide a lot of flavor; in this recipe, just over a tablespoon per serving does the job.

PER SERVING

calories 285	cholesterol 5 mg	protein 17 g	dietary exchanges
total fat 2.0 g	sodium 248 mg	calcium 91 mg	3 starch
saturated 0.5 g	carbohydrates 51 g	potassium 1,080 mg	1 vegetable
trans 0.0 g	fiber 16 g		1 very lean meat
polyunsaturated 0.5 g	sugars 11 g		
monounsaturated 1.0 g			

LENTIL SOUP
with Lemon

Lentils and potato provide wholesome fiber in this hearty main-dish soup. While it simmers, bake some Corn Muffins (page 286) and toss a salad with one of the vinaigrettes on pages 96–97.

SERVES 9 | 1 cup per serving

Lightly spray a stockpot with olive oil spray. Put the oil in the pot, swirling to coat the bottom. Cook the onion and garlic over medium-high heat for 3 minutes, or until the onion is soft, stirring frequently.

Stir in the broth, lentils, potato, oregano, and salt. Reduce the heat and simmer, covered, for 45 minutes, or until the lentils are soft.

Stir in the lemon juice and pepper.

Olive oil spray
- 1 teaspoon olive oil
- 1 small or medium onion, chopped
- 2 medium garlic cloves, minced
- 8 cups Vegetable Broth (page 53), commercial low-sodium vegetable broth, or water
- 2 cups dried lentils, sorted for stones and shriveled lentils, rinsed, and drained
- 1 medium potato, diced
- ½ teaspoon dried oregano, crumbled
- ¼ teaspoon salt
- 2 to 3 tablespoons fresh lemon juice

Pepper to taste

PER SERVING

calories 181
total fat 1.0 g
  saturated 0.0 g
  trans 0.0 g
  polyunsaturated 0.5 g
  monounsaturated 0.5 g

cholesterol 0 mg
sodium 89 mg
carbohydrates 31 g
  fiber 13 g
  sugars 2 g

protein 12 g
calcium 34 mg
potassium 523 mg

dietary exchanges
1 starch
1 very lean meat

SALADS & SALAD DRESSINGS

SPRING GREENS with Fruit, Goat Cheese, and Cranberry-Orange Vinaigrette

Use seasonal fruit so you can serve this salad with its mildly sweet and tart dressing year-round.

SERVES 4 | 2 cups salad per serving

In a shallow serving dish, arrange the salad greens, strawberries, and onion.

In a small bowl, whisk together the dressing ingredients. Pour over the salad.

Sprinkle the goat cheese on the salad. Serve immediately for the best texture.

7 ounces mixed spring greens (about 6 cups packed)

1½ cups quartered hulled strawberries or sliced apples

¼ cup thinly sliced red onion

DRESSING

⅓ cup sweetened cranberry juice

2 tablespoons honey

1½ tablespoons balsamic vinegar

1 teaspoon grated orange zest

½ teaspoon ground cumin

½ teaspoon ground cinnamon

¼ cup soft goat cheese, crumbled

PER SERVING

calories 101	**cholesterol** 3 mg	**protein** 3 g	**dietary exchanges**
total fat 2.0 g	**sodium** 42 mg	**calcium** 57 mg	½ fruit
saturated 1.0 g	**carbohydrates** 20 g	**potassium** 284 mg	1 other carbohydrate
trans 0.0 g	fiber 3 g		½ fat
polyunsaturated 0.0 g	sugars 16 g		
monounsaturated 0.5 g			

GARDEN COLESLAW

Because it doesn't contain mayonnaise, this slaw is a good picnic dish. It keeps well in the refrigerator for several days, so you can make it in advance.

SERVES 7 | ½ cup per serving

In a large bowl, toss together the slaw ingredients.

In a small bowl, whisk together the dressing ingredients. Pour over the slaw. Toss gently to coat. Cover and refrigerate for at least 1 hour before serving so the flavors blend.

SLAW

- 10 ounces shredded cabbage (8 to 9 cups)
- ½ cup chopped onion
- ½ large green bell pepper, cut into thin strips and coarsely chopped
- 1 medium carrot, shredded

DRESSING

- 3 tablespoons sugar
- 3 tablespoons white vinegar
- 2½ tablespoons water
- 1½ tablespoons canola or corn oil
- Pepper to taste

PER SERVING

calories 70	**cholesterol** 0 mg	**protein** 1 g	**dietary exchanges**
total fat 3.0 g	**sodium** 16 mg	**calcium** 24 mg	1 vegetable
saturated 0.5 g	**carbohydrates** 11 g	**potassium** 139 mg	½ other carbohydrate
trans 0.0 g	fiber 2 g		½ fat
polyunsaturated 1.0 g	sugars 8 g		
monounsaturated 2.0 g			

CUCUMBER RAITA

Serve this delightful Indian-inspired raita (*RI-tah*) to cool down a spicy entrée or use it to top Wine-Poached Salmon (page 109).

SERVES 4 | heaping ½ cup per serving

In a medium bowl, whisk together the yogurt and cayenne until the yogurt is smooth.

Stir in the cucumber and green onion. Cover and refrigerate for up to 2 hours before serving.

1½ cups fat-free plain yogurt

⅛ teaspoon cayenne

1 medium cucumber, peeled, seeded, and finely diced (about 2 cups)

1 medium green onion, finely chopped

COOK'S TIP ON ENGLISH CUCUMBERS Long and slender, English (or hothouse) cucumbers have thin skin and are virtually seedless. You can substitute one of them for the two regular cucumbers in this recipe and skip the peeling and seeding steps. English cucumbers are sold tightly wrapped in plastic. The cucumbers will keep longer if you remove the plastic before refrigerating them.

PER SERVING

calories 60	**cholesterol** 2 mg	**protein** 6 g	**dietary exchanges**
total fat 0.5 g	**sodium** 73 mg	**calcium** 190 mg	½ fat-free milk
saturated 0.0 g	**carbohydrates** 9 g	**potassium** 321 mg	
trans 0.0 g	fiber 1 g		
polyunsaturated 0.0 g	sugars 8 g		
monounsaturated 0.0 g			

TOMATO-ARTICHOKE TOSS

A sprinkling of crumbled feta tops this very tasty mix of fresh spinach, sweet grape tomatoes, artichokes, and basil.

SERVES 6 | ½ cup per serving

In a large bowl, toss together all the ingredients except the feta. Sprinkle with the feta.

7 ounces grape tomatoes, halved (about 1½ cups)

1 ounce spinach, coarsely chopped (about 1 cup)

½ 14-ounce can quartered artichoke hearts, rinsed, drained, and coarsely chopped

¼ cup finely chopped red onion

¼ cup chopped fresh basil (about ⅓ ounce)

2 tablespoons balsamic vinegar

½ teaspoon sugar

¼ teaspoon pepper

⅛ teaspoon crushed red pepper flakes (optional)

3 tablespoons crumbled low-fat feta cheese

PER SERVING

calories 33	**cholesterol** 2 mg	**protein** 2 g	**dietary exchanges**
total fat 0.5 g	**sodium** 124 mg	**calcium** 25 mg	1 vegetable
saturated 0.5 g	**carbohydrates** 6 g	**potassium** 176 mg	
trans 0.0 g	fiber 1 g		
polyunsaturated 0.0 g	sugars 3 g		
monounsaturated 0.0 g			

BALSAMIC-MARINATED VEGETABLES

This pretty, quick-to-prepare, and divine-tasting salad is perfect for potlucks and summer lunches. Vary the vegetables and try other vinaigrettes in this chapter (pages 96–97) for different flavors.

SERVES 10 | ½ cup per serving

In a large bowl, toss together the salad ingredients.

In a small bowl, whisk together the dressing ingredients. Pour over the salad, tossing well. Cover and refrigerate for 6 to 24 hours, stirring occasionally.

COOK'S TIP Vinegar-based dressings make great no-sodium or low-sodium marinades for beef, seafood, poultry, and vegetables to be grilled or broiled.

SALAD
- 1½ cups diced broccoli florets
- 1½ cups diced cauliflower florets
- 1 medium zucchini, sliced
- 12 baby carrots, sliced
- ½ cup matchstick-size slices yellow onion

DRESSING
- ½ cup water
- ¼ cup plus 2 tablespoons balsamic vinegar
- ¼ cup finely snipped fresh parsley
- 2 tablespoons canola or corn oil
- ½ teaspoon pepper

PER SERVING

calories 52	**cholesterol** 0 mg	**protein** 1 g	**dietary exchanges**
total fat 3.0 g	**sodium** 24 mg	**calcium** 22 mg	1 vegetable
saturated 0.0 g	**carbohydrates** 6 g	**potassium** 193 mg	½ fat
trans 0.0 g	fiber 2 g		
polyunsaturated 1.0 g	sugars 4 g		
monounsaturated 2.0 g			

SLICED MANGO
with Creamy Orange Sauce

A tangy yogurt-based orange sauce and a drizzle of raspberry spread dress up mango slices for an attractive dish that is terrific as a salad or a dessert.

SERVES 4 | ½ cup mango slices, 2 tablespoons sauce, and 1½ teaspoons fruit-spread mixture per serving

In a small bowl, whisk together the sauce ingredients. Set aside.

Put the fruit spread in a small microwaveable bowl. Microwave on 100 percent power (high) for 20 to 30 seconds, or until partially melted. Stir in the cinnamon. Let stand to cool slightly.

Decoratively fan the mango slices on small plates. Spoon the sauce in the center of each serving. Drizzle the fruit spread mixture over all.

SAUCE

⅓ cup fat-free plain yogurt

1 tablespoon plus 1 teaspoon fresh orange juice

Scant ½ teaspoon honey

2 tablespoons all-fruit seedless raspberry spread

¼ teaspoon ground cinnamon

1 large mango, sliced, or 2 cups sliced nectarines or peeled peaches

PER SERVING

calories 71	**cholesterol** 0 mg	**protein** 2 g	**dietary exchanges**
total fat 0.0 g	**sodium** 17 mg	**calcium** 49 mg	1 fruit
saturated 0.0 g	**carbohydrates** 17 g	**potassium** 145 mg	
trans 0.0 g	fiber 1 g		
polyunsaturated 0.0 g	sugars 14 g		
monounsaturated 0.0 g			

GRANNY APPLE AND CRANBERRY SALAD

Refreshing and crunchy, this fruit salad makes a good brunch dish with Turkey Sausage Patties (page 166).

SERVES 6 | ½ cup per serving

In a medium bowl, stir together all the ingredients. Serve immediately for peak flavor.

COOK'S TIP You can chop the apples up to 2 hours in advance. Stir in 1 to 2 teaspoons of fresh lemon juice to keep them from turning brown.

2 medium Granny Smith apples, cut into ¼-inch cubes (about 1½ cups)

½ cup sweetened dried cranberries

½ teaspoon grated orange zest

¼ cup fresh orange juice

2 tablespoons chopped pecans, dry-roasted

¼ teaspoon ground cinnamon

PER SERVING

calories 85	**cholesterol** 0 mg	**protein** 0 g	**dietary exchanges**
total fat 2.0 g	**sodium** 1 mg	**calcium** 8 mg	1 fruit
saturated 0.0 g	**carbohydrates** 18 g	**potassium** 100 mg	½ fat
trans 0.0 g	fiber 2 g		
polyunsaturated 0.5 g	sugars 15 g		
monounsaturated 1.0 g			

SUMMER PASTA SALAD

Crisp, colorful vegetables are the highlights of this salad. Try it for a summertime picnic for a group or for the next family reunion.

SERVES 10 | ½ cup per serving

In a stockpot, prepare the pasta using the package directions, omitting the salt. When the pasta has boiled for 4 minutes, stir in the broccoli and carrots. Boil for 1 minute.

Stir in the squash. Boil for 30 seconds. Immediately transfer the pasta mixture to a colander. Run under cold water to stop the cooking process and cool quickly. Drain well. Set aside.

In a large bowl, whisk together the dressing ingredients.

Add the pasta mixture to the dressing. Toss gently to coat. Sprinkle with the Parmesan and salt. Toss gently. Cover and refrigerate for 15 minutes to 4 hours before serving.

4 ounces dried whole-grain rotini (about 1½ cups)

1½ cups broccoli florets

½ cup sliced carrots, cut on the diagonal

1 cup sliced yellow summer squash

DRESSING

3 tablespoons chopped fresh basil or 1 tablespoon dried, crumbled

3 tablespoons cider vinegar

1 tablespoon olive oil (extra virgin preferred)

2 medium garlic cloves, minced

¼ teaspoon pepper

2 tablespoons shredded or grated Parmesan cheese

⅛ teaspoon salt

COOK'S TIP ON EXTRA-VIRGIN OLIVE OIL

Extra-virgin olive oil is considered to be the fruitiest of all olive oils. It is available in a variety of shades from crystalline to bright green. For a more intense olive flavor, choose an oil that is deeper in color.

PER SERVING

calories 67	**cholesterol** 1 mg	**protein** 3 g	**dietary exchanges**
total fat 2.0 g	**sodium** 56 mg	**calcium** 30 mg	½ starch
saturated 0.5 g	**carbohydrates** 11 g	**potassium** 126 mg	
trans 0.0 g	fiber 2 g		
polyunsaturated 0.0 g	sugars 1 g		
monounsaturated 1.0 g			

MEDITERRANEAN COUSCOUS

Couscous, a quick-cooking Moroccan staple, gets a Mediterranean makeover with fresh lemon juice, oregano, mint, and feta.

SERVES 8 | ½ cup per serving

Prepare the couscous using the package directions, omitting the salt. Fluff with a fork. Set aside to cool.

Meanwhile, in a medium bowl, stir together the remaining ingredients except the feta. Gently stir in the cooled couscous. Sprinkle with the feta. Serve immediately for peak flavor.

⅓ cup uncooked whole-wheat couscous

8 ounces frozen artichoke quarters, thawed, drained, and chopped

1 large Italian plum (Roma) tomato, chopped

½ medium cucumber, peeled and diced

2 tablespoons finely chopped red onion

2 tablespoons snipped fresh parsley

2 tablespoons fresh lemon juice

1 tablespoon chopped fresh oregano or 1 teaspoon dried, crumbled

1 tablespoon minced fresh mint or 1 teaspoon dried, crumbled

1 tablespoon olive oil (extra virgin preferred)

½ teaspoon garlic powder

3 tablespoons crumbled feta cheese

CILANTRO COUSCOUS

SERVES 8 | ½ cup per serving

Prepare the couscous using the package directions, omitting the salt. Fluff with a fork. Set aside to cool.

Meanwhile, in a medium bowl, stir together the remaining ingredients. Gently stir in the cooled couscous. Serve immediately for peak flavor.

⅓ cup uncooked whole-wheat couscous

8 ounces frozen artichoke quarters, thawed, drained, and chopped

1 large Italian plum (Roma) tomato, chopped

½ medium cucumber, peeled and diced

½ 2.25-ounce can sliced black olives, drained

2 tablespoons finely chopped radish

2 tablespoons snipped fresh parsley

2 tablespoons snipped fresh cilantro

2 tablespoons fresh lemon juice

1 tablespoon olive oil (extra virgin preferred)

½ teaspoon garlic powder

2 to 3 drops red hot-pepper sauce, or to taste (optional)

PER SERVING

calories 94	**cholesterol** 6 mg	**protein** 4 g	**dietary exchanges**
total fat 4.0 g	**sodium** 108 mg	**calcium** 56 mg	½ starch
saturated 1.5 g	**carbohydrates** 12 g	**potassium** 156 mg	1 vegetable
trans 0.0 g	fiber 3 g		1 fat
polyunsaturated 0.5 g	sugars 1 g		
monounsaturated 1.5 g			

PER SERVING
CILANTRO COUSCOUS

calories 79	**cholesterol** 0 mg	**protein** 3 g	**dietary exchanges**
total fat 3.0 g	**sodium** 87 mg	**calcium** 22 mg	½ starch
saturated 0.5 g	**carbohydrates** 12 g	**potassium** 144 mg	1 vegetable
trans 0.0 g	fiber 3 g		1 fat
polyunsaturated 0.5 g	sugars 1 g		
monounsaturated 2.0 g			

COUSCOUS
with Walnuts and Dried Fruit

A just-right blend of sweet and tart, this salad is a great accompaniment to Curried Chicken Kebabs with Yogurt Dipping Sauce (page 138) or Pork Chops with Herb Rub (page 196). Spoon the salad onto leaves of butter lettuce or radicchio for an especially attractive presentation.

SERVES 4 | ¾ cup per serving

In a medium saucepan, bring the water just to a boil. Stir in the couscous. Remove from the heat and let stand, covered, for 5 minutes. Lightly fluff with a fork

Meanwhile, in a medium bowl, whisk together the lime zest, lime juice, cumin, and garlic. Whisk in the oil.

Add the couscous, tossing gently. Add the remaining ingredients, tossing gently. Serve at room temperature.

1¼ cups water

¾ cup uncooked whole-wheat couscous

Grated zest of 1 medium lime

3 tablespoons fresh lime juice

½ teaspoon ground cumin

1 medium garlic clove, minced

2 tablespoons olive oil (extra virgin preferred)

1 medium red bell pepper, diced

1 medium green onion, finely chopped

8 dried apricot halves, diced

3 tablespoons golden raisins

2 tablespoons snipped fresh cilantro

2 tablespoons chopped walnuts, dry-roasted

⅛ teaspoon pepper

PER SERVING

calories 298	**cholesterol** 0 mg	**protein** 8 g	**dietary exchanges**
total fat 10.0 g	**sodium** 8 mg	**calcium** 37 mg	2 starch
saturated 1.5 g	**carbohydrates** 49 g	**potassium** 315 mg	1 fruit
trans 0.0 g	fiber 7 g		1½ fat
polyunsaturated 3.0 g	sugars 10 g		
monounsaturated 5.5 g			

SOUTHWESTERN BLACK-EYED PEA SALAD

A popular dish in the Lone Star State, where it is called Texas Caviar, this flavorful salad is sure to become a favorite in your household, too.

SERVES 10 | ½ cup per serving

In a medium bowl, stir together all the ingredients except the peas. Stir in the peas. Cover and refrigerate for 2 to 24 hours before serving.

COOK'S TIP ON HOT CHILE PEPPERS Hot chile peppers, such as jalapeño, Anaheim, serrano, and poblano, contain oils that can burn your skin, lips, and eyes. Wear plastic gloves or wash your hands thoroughly with warm, soapy water immediately after handling hot peppers. Most of the spicy heat in a chile pepper, such as the jalapeño in this salad, is found in the seeds and ribs (membranes). Leave them in for maximum heat, or discard them if you prefer a milder flavor.

½ medium green bell pepper, diced

1 small white onion, diced

3 tablespoons red wine vinegar

2 tablespoons finely chopped fresh jalapeño, seeds and ribs discarded

1 tablespoon canola or corn oil

1 tablespoon water

1 medium garlic clove, minced

¼ teaspoon pepper

3 15.5-ounce cans no-salt-added black-eyed peas, rinsed and drained, or 3 10-ounce packages frozen black-eyed peas, cooked

PER SERVING

calories 131
total fat 1.5 g
  saturated 0.0 g
  trans 0.0 g
  polyunsaturated 0.5 g
  monounsaturated 1.0 g

cholesterol 0 mg
sodium 1 mg
carbohydrates 22 g
  fiber 5 g
  sugars 5 g

protein 7 g
calcium 43 mg
potassium 327 mg

dietary exchanges
1½ starch
½ very lean meat

ASIAN BROWN RICE AND VEGETABLE SALAD

This main-dish salad, topped with a sesame-wasabi dressing, is an interesting combination of colors, textures, aromas, and flavors.

SERVES 4 | ½ cup rice, ½ cup spinach, ½ cup broccoli slaw, and 2 tablespoons dressing per serving

In a medium saucepan, stir together the water, 2 tablespoons vinegar, brown sugar, and gingerroot. Bring to a simmer over medium-high heat, stirring occasionally.

Stir in the rice. Reduce the heat and simmer, covered, for 10 minutes. Remove the pan from the heat. Let stand, covered, for 5 minutes. Fluff the rice with a fork. Let the mixture cool in the pan, uncovered, for 5 to 10 minutes.

Meanwhile, in a small bowl, whisk together the broth, remaining 1 tablespoon vinegar, soy sauce, oil, and wasabi. Set aside.

For each serving, make a single layer of spinach on a salad plate, followed in order by a layer each of rice, broccoli slaw, and walnuts. Drizzle about 2 tablespoons of dressing over each salad.

1¼ cups water

2 tablespoons plain rice or white wine vinegar and 1 tablespoon plain rice or white wine vinegar, divided use

1 tablespoon light brown sugar

1 teaspoon grated peeled gingerroot

1 cup uncooked instant brown rice

⅓ cup Chicken Broth (page 50) or commercial fat-free, low-sodium chicken broth

2 teaspoons soy sauce (lowest sodium available)

1 teaspoon toasted sesame oil

½ teaspoon wasabi paste

2 ounces spinach (about 2 cups)

2 cups broccoli slaw

2 tablespoons chopped walnuts, dry-roasted

COOK'S TIP ON WASABI Add *small* amounts of wasabi paste to various dishes, such as salad dressings, marinades, and sauces, to enhance the flavor without adding sodium. Just proceed carefully—wasabi, sometimes called Japanese horseradish, is fiery!

COOK'S TIP ON GINGERROOT If the produce section of your grocery store has only large pieces of gingerroot, it is appropriate to break off what you need. Use a spoon, knife, or vegetable peeler to remove the skin before grating, slicing, or finely chopping the flesh.

PER SERVING

calories 150	**cholesterol** 0 mg	**protein** 4 g	**dietary exchanges**
total fat 4.5 g	**sodium** 110 mg	**calcium** 24 mg	1½ starch
saturated 0.5 g	**carbohydrates** 24 g	**potassium** 248 mg	½ fat
trans 0.0 g	fiber 3 g		
polyunsaturated 2.5 g	sugars 4 g		
monounsaturated 1.0 g			

RED-POTATO SALAD

The right amount of mustard is a key ingredient for great potato salad. Since yellow mustard is usually high in sodium, this recipe calls for dry mustard instead.

SERVES 9 | ½ cup per serving

In a large bowl, stir together the salad ingredients.

In a small bowl, whisk together the dressing ingredients. Pour into the potato mixture, stirring gently to coat. Cover and refrigerate for about 2 hours before serving.

SALAD

1½ to 2 pounds red potatoes, cooked and diced

1 or 2 medium ribs of celery, chopped

6 medium radishes, sliced

2 medium green onions, sliced

DRESSING

3 tablespoons fat-free sour cream

2½ tablespoons vinegar

2 tablespoons light mayonnaise

2 tablespoons fat-free plain yogurt

1 tablespoon sugar

1 teaspoon dry mustard

½ teaspoon celery seeds (optional)

¼ teaspoon pepper

¼ teaspoon turmeric

PER SERVING

calories 92
total fat 1.0 g
  saturated 0.0 g
  trans 0.0 g
  polyunsaturated 0.5 g
  monounsaturated 0.0 g

cholesterol 2 mg
sodium 43 mg
carbohydrates 19 g
  fiber 2 g
  sugars 3 g

protein 3 g
calcium 34 mg
potassium 434 mg

dietary exchanges
1½ starch

SALMON AND CUCUMBER SALAD with Basil-Lime Dressing

The combination of fresh basil and lime in the dressing makes this dish distinctive and delightful. It's a nice and easy way to work some fish into your week.

SERVES 4 | 1½ cups salad greens and scant 1 cup salmon salad per serving

In a medium bowl, whisk together the lime zest, lime juice, and pepper. Slowly whisk in the oil. Stir in the basil. Set aside 2 tablespoons of the dressing in a large bowl.

Add the salmon salad ingredients to the dressing remaining in the medium bowl, tossing gently to coat. Set aside.

Add the salad greens to the 2 tablespoons dressing in the large bowl, tossing to coat. Arrange the salad greens on plates. Spoon the salmon salad over the salad greens.

DRESSING

- 1 teaspoon grated lime zest
- 2 tablespoons fresh lime juice
- ⅛ teaspoon pepper
- 2 tablespoons olive oil (extra virgin preferred)
- 2 tablespoons chopped fresh basil

SALMON SALAD

- 2 5-ounce vacuum-sealed pouches pink salmon, flaked
- 1 cup diced seeded cucumber (English, or hothouse, preferred)
- 1 cup grape tomatoes, halved
- ½ cup diced red bell pepper

- 6 ounces mixed salad greens (about 6 cups; baby greens preferred)

PER SERVING

calories 194	**cholesterol** 58 mg	**protein** 19 g	**dietary exchanges**
total fat 10.5 g	**sodium** 311 mg	**calcium** 254 mg	2 vegetable
saturated 1.5 g	**carbohydrates** 8 g	**potassium** 700 mg	2½ lean meat
trans 0.0 g	fiber 3 g		1 fat
polyunsaturated 2.0 g	sugars 4 g		
monounsaturated 5.5 g			

TROPICAL TUNA SALAD

A scoop of crunchy tuna salad on a bed of juicy mango slices makes a nice lunch entrée.

SERVES 4 | ¼ cup tuna salad and scant ½ cup mango slices per serving

Arrange the mango slices on salad plates.

In a medium bowl, stir together the salad ingredients. Using a small ice-cream scoop or spoon, mound the tuna salad on the mango slices.

COOK'S TIP To complete the presentation of this salad, add a colorful, fragrant—and edible—garnish of sprigs of fresh herbs. Some good choices are mint, basil, rosemary, thyme, tarragon, lemon balm, or lavender.

1 medium mango, sliced, or 1½ cups sliced bottled mango, drained

SALAD

1 5-ounce can very low sodium albacore tuna packed in water, drained and flaked

½ cup pineapple tidbits canned in their own juice, drained

¼ medium carrot, shredded

2 tablespoons light mayonnaise

2 tablespoons chopped walnuts, dry-roasted

½ teaspoon grated lemon zest

2 teaspoons fresh lemon juice

⅛ teaspoon pepper

PER SERVING

calories 137	**cholesterol** 17 mg	**protein** 9 g	**dietary exchanges**
total fat 5.5 g	**sodium** 90 mg	**calcium** 16 mg	1 fruit
saturated 0.5 g	**carbohydrates** 15 g	**potassium** 222 mg	1½ lean meat
trans 0.0 g	fiber 2 g		
polyunsaturated 3.5 g	sugars 12 g		
monounsaturated 1.0 g			

CHICKEN SALAD

Celery and green onions give this versatile salad a crunch and a fresh taste that will make you want to use it as often as you can—to stuff a tomato, fill half a pita, or provide protein on a salad plate.

SERVES 5 | ½ cup per serving

In a medium bowl, stir together the chicken, celery, and green onions.

In a small bowl, whisk together the remaining ingredients. Pour over the chicken mixture, stirring to combine. Serve immediately or cover and refrigerate until needed.

COOK'S TIP Garnish this salad with halved seedless grapes, pineapple chunks, Sweet Bread-and-Butter Pickles (page 274), or tomato wedges.

3 5-ounce cans no-salt-added chicken breast, packed in water, drained and shredded

1 medium rib of celery, finely chopped

4 medium green onions, chopped

½ cup light mayonnaise

½ teaspoon Dijon mustard (lowest sodium available)

¼ teaspoon ground ginger

¼ teaspoon pepper

PER SERVING

calories 158	**cholesterol** 46 mg	**protein** 18 g	**dietary exchanges**
total fat 7.0 g	**sodium** 282 mg	**calcium** 4 mg	2½ lean meat
saturated 0.5 g	**carbohydrates** 4 g	**potassium** 197 mg	
trans 0.0 g	fiber 1 g		
polyunsaturated 4.5 g	sugars 1 g		
monounsaturated 2.0 g			

MEXICAN QUINOA AND CHICKEN SALAD

This salad gets its flavor from cumin, jalapeño, lime juice—and, surprisingly, a touch of honey.

SERVES 4 | 1½ cups per serving

In a medium saucepan, combine the quinoa and 1 cup water. Bring to a boil, covered, over medium-high heat. Reduce the heat and simmer, still covered, for 12 minutes.

Stir in the corn. Simmer, covered, for 3 to 4 minutes, or until the water is absorbed, the quinoa is translucent and tender, and the corn is crisp-tender. Remove from the heat. Set aside.

In a small bowl, whisk together the lime juice, cilantro, oil, cumin, pepper, honey, and remaining 2 tablespoons water. Set aside.

In a salad bowl, toss together the chicken, bell pepper, tomatoes, green onions, and jalapeño. Add the quinoa mixture, tossing to combine. Drizzle with the lime juice mixture, tossing to combine.

Place the lettuce leaves on plates. Spoon the salad onto the lettuce.

½ cup uncooked prerinsed quinoa

1 cup water and 2 tablespoons water, divided use

1 cup fresh or frozen corn, thawed if frozen

⅓ cup fresh lime juice

2 tablespoons snipped fresh cilantro

1 teaspoon olive oil

½ teaspoon ground cumin

¼ teaspoon pepper

¼ teaspoon honey

1 pound boneless, skinless chicken breasts, cooked without salt, all visible fat discarded, cubed

1 medium red bell pepper, finely chopped

½ cup grape tomatoes, halved

2 medium green onions, sliced

1 medium fresh jalapeño, seeds and ribs discarded, diced

4 large lettuce leaves

COOK'S TIP ON QUINOA Mildly flavored and high in protein, quinoa is nutritious and cooks quickly. Try it in place of rice or couscous in recipes or as a side dish. Often called a supergrain, quinoa is covered with a bitter-tasting coating of saponin, a harmless naturally occurring substance. If the quinoa is not prerinsed, put it in a fine-mesh sieve and rinse it under cold running water to be sure to get rid of the coating.

PER SERVING

calories 277	**cholesterol** 66 mg	**protein** 31 g	**dietary exchanges**
total fat 4.5 g	**sodium** 91 mg	**calcium** 38 mg	1½ starch
saturated 1.0 g	**carbohydrates** 28 g	**potassium** 732 mg	1 vegetable
trans 0.0 g	fiber 4 g		3 very lean meat
polyunsaturated 1.5 g	sugars 5 g		
monounsaturated 1.5 g			

PACIFIC RIM STEAK SALAD
with Sweet-and-Sour Dressing

Dinner is on the table in minutes when Pacific Rim Flank Steak (page 180) or other cooked steak becomes part of this entrée salad.

SERVES 4 | 1½ cups salad, 2 ounces beef, and 2 tablespoons dressing per serving

Cook the edamame using the package directions, omitting the salt. Drain well in a colander.

Meanwhile, in a small bowl, whisk together the pineapple juice, sweet-and-sour sauce, and oil. Set aside.

Arrange the lettuce on plates. Top with the edamame and remaining ingredients. Pour 2 tablespoons dressing over each serving.

COOK'S TIP ON SESAME OIL Sesame oil comes from sesame seeds; the darker variety of oil, often called toasted sesame oil, is made from toasted sesame seeds and has a more robust flavor and aroma than regular sesame oil. It takes only a small amount of toasted sesame oil to add a lot of flavor.

½ cup frozen shelled edamame (green soybeans)

¾ cup pineapple juice

2 tablespoons Chinese sweet-and-sour sauce (lowest sodium available)

⅛ teaspoon toasted sesame oil

4 ounces romaine or lettuce blend with romaine, torn into bite-size pieces (about 4 cups)

8 ounces flank steak cooked without salt (such as from Pacific Rim Flank Steak), thinly sliced on the diagonal, warmed if desired

1 cup fresh pineapple chunks or pineapple chunks canned in their own juice, drained

½ large red bell pepper, sliced lengthwise

2 medium crosswise slices of red onion, separated into rings

PER SERVING

calories 226	**cholesterol** 40 mg	**protein** 22 g	**dietary exchanges**
total fat 6.5 g	**sodium** 45 mg	**calcium** 37 mg	1 fruit
saturated 2.5 g	**carbohydrates** 19 g	**potassium** 531 mg	1 vegetable
trans 0.0 g	fiber 3 g		2 lean meat
polyunsaturated 0.5 g	sugars 13 g		
monounsaturated 3.0 g			

SESAME-GINGER DRESSING

Green tea on your salad? Yes, it makes a great base for this Asian-style dressing, which lets you duplicate the flavor of restaurant salads at home without all the extra salt. Toss the dressing with a variety of salad greens and raw vegetables for a side salad or add grilled chicken, shrimp, or lean beef strips for an entrée.

SERVES 4 | 2 tablespoons per serving

Pour the boiling water into a small bowl or other container that will hold at least 1 cup of liquid. Add the tea bag and let it steep for 1 minute. Discard the tea bag. Let the tea cool for 10 to 15 minutes.

Whisk in the remaining ingredients. If not using right away, cover and refrigerate for up to three days.

⅓ cup boiling water

1 single-serving bag of green tea

2 tablespoons plain rice vinegar

1 tablespoon dry-roasted sesame seeds

1 teaspoon minced peeled gingerroot

1 medium garlic clove, minced

½ teaspoon toasted sesame oil

PER SERVING

calories 22	**cholesterol** 0 mg	**protein** 1 g	**dietary exchanges**
total fat 2.0 g	**sodium** 2 mg	**calcium** 3 mg	½ fat
saturated 0.5 g	**carbohydrates** 1 g	**potassium** 21 mg	
trans 0.0 g	fiber 0 g		
polyunsaturated 1.0 g	sugars 0 g		
monounsaturated 1.0 g			

CIDER VINAIGRETTE

Fresh lemon juice and garlic intensify the flavor of this dressing. You'll be able to complement many different types of salad with it and its variations.

SERVES 8 | 2 tablespoons per serving

In a small bowl, whisk together all the ingredients. Cover and refrigerate until needed.

For each variation below, follow the same instructions.

⅓ cup cider vinegar

¼ cup fresh lemon juice

3 tablespoons water

2 tablespoons canola or corn oil

1½ tablespoons Dijon mustard (lowest sodium available)

2½ teaspoons sugar

2 medium garlic cloves, minced

½ teaspoon pepper

ITALIAN DRESSING

SERVES 8 | 2 tablespoons per serving

1 recipe Cider Vinaigrette

1 teaspoon dried basil, crumbled

1 teaspoon dried oregano, crumbled

TOMATO FRENCH DRESSING

SERVES 10 | 2 tablespoons per serving

1 recipe Cider Vinaigrette

3 tablespoons no-salt-added tomato paste

2 teaspoons sugar

1 tablespoon dehydrated minced onion

RUSSIAN DRESSING

SERVES 10 | 2 tablespoons per serving

- 1 recipe Cider Vinaigrette
- 2 tablespoons no-salt-added tomato paste
- 1 tablespoon finely chopped green bell pepper
- ¼ teaspoon Chili Powder (page 277) or no-salt-added chili powder
- ⅛ teaspoon onion powder

Dash of red hot-pepper sauce

PER SERVING

calories 45
total fat 3.5 g
  saturated 0.5 g
  trans 0.0 g
  polyunsaturated 1.0 g
  monounsaturated 2.0 g

cholesterol 0 mg
sodium 59 mg
carbohydrates 3 g
  fiber 0 g
  sugars 2 g

protein 0 g
calcium 5 mg
potassium 27 mg

dietary exchanges
1 fat

PER SERVING
ITALIAN DRESSING

calories 46
total fat 3.5 g
  saturated 0.5 g
  trans 0.0 g
  polyunsaturated 1.0 g
  monounsaturated 2.0 g

cholesterol 0 mg
sodium 59 mg
carbohydrates 3 g
  fiber 0 g
  sugars 2 g

protein 0 g
calcium 12 mg
potassium 36 mg

dietary exchanges
1 fat

PER SERVING
TOMATO FRENCH DRESSING

calories 45
total fat 3.0 g
  saturated 0.0 g
  trans 0.0 g
  polyunsaturated 1.0 g
  monounsaturated 2.0 g

cholesterol 0 mg
sodium 52 mg
carbohydrates 4 g
  fiber 0 g
  sugars 3 g

protein 1 g
calcium 7 mg
potassium 77 mg

dietary exchanges
½ fat

PER SERVING
RUSSIAN DRESSING

calories 39
total fat 3.0 g
  saturated 0.0 g
  trans 0.0 g
  polyunsaturated 1.0 g
  monounsaturated 2.0 g

cholesterol 0 mg
sodium 50 mg
carbohydrates 3 g
  fiber 0 g
  sugars 2 g

protein 0 g
calcium 6 mg
potassium 58 mg

dietary exchanges
½ fat

RANCH DRESSING
with Fresh Herbs

Fresh dillweed and parsley perk up this low-salt version of a classic.

SERVES 12 | 2 tablespoons per serving

In a small bowl, whisk together all the ingredients. Cover and refrigerate for at least 2 hours so the flavors blend.

1 cup low-fat buttermilk

½ cup fat-free sour cream

1 tablespoon snipped fresh dillweed

1 tablespoon snipped fresh parsley

1 tablespoon Dijon mustard (lowest sodium available)

2 teaspoons dehydrated minced onion

¼ teaspoon garlic powder

⅛ to ¼ teaspoon pepper

PER SERVING

calories 21
total fat 0.5 g
  saturated 0.0 g
  trans 0.0 g
  polyunsaturated 0.0 g
  monounsaturated 0.0 g

cholesterol 3 mg
sodium 56 mg
carbohydrates 3 g
  fiber 0 g
  sugars 2 g

protein 2 g
calcium 46 mg
potassium 63 mg

dietary exchanges
free

THOUSAND ISLAND DRESSING

Creamy and just a wee bit spicy, this classic dressing is the finishing touch that will make your salad creations irresistible.

SERVES 10 | 2 tablespoons per serving

In a small bowl, whisk together all the ingredients. Cover and refrigerate until needed.

½ cup fat-free plain yogurt

½ cup Chili Sauce (page 276), or ½ cup no-salt-added ketchup plus dash of red hot-pepper sauce

2 tablespoons light mayonnaise

White of 1 large hard-cooked egg, finely chopped (yolk discarded)

1 tablespoon finely chopped green bell pepper

1 tablespoon finely chopped celery

¼ teaspoon onion powder

Dash of pepper

PER SERVING

calories 30
total fat 1.0 g
  saturated 0.0 g
  trans 0.0 g
  polyunsaturated 0.5 g
  monounsaturated 0.0 g

cholesterol 1 mg
sodium 47 mg
carbohydrates 4 g
  fiber 0 g
  sugars 4 g

protein 1 g
calcium 29 mg
potassium 106 mg

dietary exchanges
free

APRICOT-YOGURT DRESSING

Spoon this dressing over fresh fruit, such as melon or pineapple, when you want a pretty side salad or a light dessert.

SERVES 10 | 2 tablespoons per serving

In a small bowl, whisk together all the ingredients. Cover and refrigerate until needed.

- 1 cup fat-free plain yogurt
- ¼ cup all-fruit apricot spread
- 2 teaspoons honey
- ½ teaspoon vanilla extract

PER SERVING

calories 35
total fat 0.0 g
  saturated 0.0 g
  trans 0.0 g
  polyunsaturated 0.0 g
  monounsaturated 0.0 g

cholesterol 1 mg
sodium 19 mg
carbohydrates 7 g
  fiber 0 g
  sugars 6 g

protein 1 g
calcium 49 mg
potassium 64 mg

dietary exchanges
  ½ other carbohydrate

SEAFOOD

PAN-SEARED FILLETS
with Cilantro

Quickly sear the fish fillets, then keep them moist by reducing the heat. Top them with a mild zing of jalapeño and a splash of fresh lime—that's dinner in a snap!

SERVES 4 | 3 ounces fish per serving

In a small bowl, stir together the paprika, pepper, and salt. Sprinkle over one side of each fillet. Using your fingertips, gently press the mixture so it adheres to the fish.

Heat a large nonstick skillet over medium-high heat. Cook the fish with the seasoned side down for 2 minutes. Reduce the heat to medium. Turn the fish over. Cook for 4 to 5 minutes, or until it flakes easily when tested with a fork. Remove from the heat.

Meanwhile, in another small bowl, stir together the jalapeño, cilantro, and margarine. Using the back of a spoon, spread the jalapeño mixture over the seasoned side of the fish. Squeeze the lime over the fish. Serve with the seasoned side up.

½ teaspoon paprika

¼ teaspoon pepper

¼ teaspoon salt

4 mild white fish fillets (about 4 ounces each), rinsed and patted dry

½ medium fresh jalapeño, seeds and ribs discarded, minced

2 tablespoons snipped fresh cilantro

2 tablespoons light tub margarine

1 medium lime, cut into 4 wedges

PER SERVING

calories 129	**cholesterol** 42 mg	**protein** 22 g	**dietary exchanges**
total fat 3.5 g	**sodium** 251 mg	**calcium** 34 mg	3 very lean meat
saturated 0.5 g	**carbohydrates** 1 g	**potassium** 578 mg	
trans 0.0 g	fiber 0 g		
polyunsaturated 1.0 g	sugars 0 g		
monounsaturated 1.5 g			

SPICY BAKED FISH

A crust of whole-wheat crumbs and snipped fresh parsley with just a few drops of hot-pepper sauce kicks up the flavor of mild fish.

SERVES 4 | 3 ounces fish per serving

Preheat the oven to 350°F.

Sprinkle the bread crumbs on an ungreased baking sheet.

Bake for 5 to 7 minutes, or until lightly browned.

Meanwhile, in a medium shallow dish, whisk together the mayonnaise, water, and hot-pepper sauce. Set aside.

Transfer the bread crumbs to a separate medium shallow dish. Stir in the parsley and pepper.

Increase the oven temperature to 450°F.

Lightly spray the same baking sheet with cooking spray. Set the shallow dishes and the baking sheet in a row, assembly-line fashion. Dip a fillet in the mayonnaise mixture, turning to coat. Dip in the bread crumb mixture, turning to coat and gently shaking off any excess. Transfer to the baking sheet. Repeat with the remaining fillets.

Bake for 17 to 18 minutes, or until the fish flakes easily when tested with a fork. Serve with the lemon wedges to squeeze over the fish.

2 slices light whole-wheat bread (lowest sodium available), processed to very fine crumbs

2 tablespoons light mayonnaise

1 tablespoon water

4 drops red hot-pepper sauce

¼ cup snipped fresh parsley

½ teaspoon pepper

Cooking spray

4 mild white fish fillets (about 4 ounces each), rinsed and patted dry

1 medium lemon, cut into 4 wedges (optional)

PER SERVING

calories 122	**cholesterol** 46 mg	**protein** 19 g	**dietary exchanges**
total fat 2.5 g	**sodium** 186 mg	**calcium** 27 mg	½ starch
saturated 0.5 g	**carbohydrates** 5 g	**potassium** 240 mg	3 very lean meat
trans 0.0 g	fiber 2 g		
polyunsaturated 1.5 g	sugars 1 g		
monounsaturated 0.5 g			

MEDITERRANEAN FISH FILLETS

Fresh lemon juice, capers, basil, and olive oil provide your palate with a taste from the Greek Isles.

SERVES 6 | 3 ounces fish per serving

Preheat the oven to 350°F. Lightly spray a rimmed baking sheet with olive oil spray.

Place the fish in a single layer on the baking sheet. Drizzle with the lemon juice. Sprinkle with the pepper. Top with the tomatoes, bell pepper, and capers.

In a small bowl, stir together the bread crumbs, oil, and basil. Sprinkle over the fish.

Bake for 25 minutes, or until the fish flakes easily when tested with a fork.

COOK'S TIP ON MILD WHITE FISH Factors including taste preference, availability, freshness, price, and avoidance of what is being overharvested may affect your choice of mild white fish. Many varieties, such as cod, grouper, haddock, mahimahi, sea bass, scrod, sole, and tilapia, are interchangeable, needing only minor adjustments in cooking time to account for differences in thickness.

Olive oil spray

6 mild white fish fillets (about 4 ounces each), rinsed and patted dry

Juice of 1 medium lemon

⅛ teaspoon pepper

2 large tomatoes, sliced ¼ inch thick

½ medium green bell pepper, finely chopped

2 tablespoons capers packed in balsamic vinegar, drained

¼ cup plain dry bread crumbs (lowest sodium available)

1 tablespoon olive oil

1½ teaspoons dried basil, crumbled

PER SERVING

calories 136	**cholesterol** 43 mg	**protein** 19 g	**dietary exchanges**
total fat 3.5 g	**sodium** 183 mg	**calcium** 36 mg	½ starch
saturated 0.5 g	**carbohydrates** 7 g	**potassium** 385 mg	3 very lean meat
trans 0.0 g	fiber 1 g		
polyunsaturated 0.5 g	sugars 2 g		
monounsaturated 2.0 g			

SOUTHERN FISH FILLETS

Pair this cornmeal-coated fish with Garden Coleslaw (page 75) and Green Beans and Corn (page 236) for a healthy southern meal.

SERVES 4 | 3 ounces fish per serving

Preheat the oven to 450°F. Lightly spray a 13 x 9 x 2-inch glass baking dish with cooking spray. Set aside.

In a medium shallow dish, stir together the milk and hot-pepper sauce.

In a separate medium shallow dish, stir together the cornmeal, parsley, tarragon, pepper, and cayenne.

Set the shallow dishes and baking dish in a row, assembly-line fashion. Dip a fillet in the milk mixture, turning to coat and letting any excess drip off. Dip in the cornmeal mixture, turning to coat and gently shaking off any excess. Transfer to the baking dish. Repeat with the remaining fillets.

Bake for 15 to 17 minutes, or until the fish flakes easily when tested with a fork. Serve with the lemon wedges to squeeze over the fish.

Cooking spray
- ½ cup fat-free milk
- 4 drops red hot-pepper sauce
- ½ cup yellow cornmeal
- ¼ cup finely snipped fresh parsley
- 1 teaspoon dried tarragon, crumbled
- ½ teaspoon pepper
- ¼ teaspoon cayenne
- 4 mild white fish fillets (about 4 ounces each), rinsed
- 1 medium lemon, cut into 4 wedges (optional)

PER SERVING

calories 162	**cholesterol** 69 mg	**protein** 21 g	**dietary exchanges**
total fat 1.0 g	**sodium** 98 mg	**calcium** 61 mg	1 starch
saturated 0.0 g	**carbohydrates** 17 g	**potassium** 302 mg	3 very lean meat
trans 0.0 g	fiber 1 g		
polyunsaturated 0.5 g	sugars 2 g		
monounsaturated 0.5 g			

PECAN-CRUSTED CATFISH
with Zesty Tartar Sauce

Sour cream replaces mayonnaise as the base for the tartar sauce here. Serve this fish with corn on the cob and chilled slices of melon on the side.

SERVES 4 | 3 ounces fish and 2 tablespoons sauce per serving

Put the fish in a single layer in a large shallow dish. Drizzle the top side with half the buttermilk, spreading to cover. Turn the fish over and repeat with the remaining buttermilk. Cover and refrigerate for 10 minutes to 1 hour, turning occasionally.

Preheat the oven to 400°F.

In a food processor or blender, process the bread for 5 to 10 seconds to make soft crumbs.

In a shallow dish, stir together the bread crumbs, green onions, pecans, and lemon pepper.

Drain the fish, discarding the buttermilk. Add the fish to the bread-crumb mixture, turning to coat. Using your fingertips, gently press the mixture so it adheres to the fish. Reserve any remaining bread-crumb mixture. Transfer the fish to a nonstick baking sheet. Sprinkle with the reserved bread-crumb mixture.

Bake for 10 to 12 minutes, or until the fish flakes easily when tested with a fork.

Meanwhile, in a small bowl, whisk together the tartar sauce ingredients. Cover and refrigerate until serving time. Serve with the fish.

FISH

- 4 catfish fillets (about 4 ounces each), rinsed
- 2 tablespoons low-fat buttermilk
- 2 slices light whole-wheat bread (lowest sodium available), coarsely torn
- 2 medium green onions, thinly sliced
- 3 tablespoons chopped pecans
- ½ teaspoon salt-free lemon pepper

TARTAR SAUCE

- ½ cup fat-free sour cream
- 2 tablespoons dill pickle relish
- 1 teaspoon grated lemon zest
- 1 teaspoon fresh lemon juice
- ½ teaspoon dried dillweed, crumbled

PER SERVING

calories 212	**cholesterol** 71 mg	**protein** 22 g	**dietary exchanges**
total fat 7.0 g	**sodium** 224 mg	**calcium** 102 mg	1 starch
saturated 1.0 g	**carbohydrates** 14 g	**potassium** 586 mg	3 lean meat
trans 0.0 g	fiber 3 g		
polyunsaturated 2.0 g	sugars 6 g		
monounsaturated 3.0 g			

MOROCCAN-STYLE HALIBUT
with Mango and Golden Raisin Relish

In less than 30 minutes from starting to prep the ingredients to serving, you can make this exotic fish dish and the accompanying fruit relish. Another time, make only the fruit relish and serve it with roasted pork or chicken.

SERVES 4 | 3 ounces fish and ¼ cup relish per serving

In a small bowl, stir together the relish ingredients. Set aside.

In another small bowl, stir together the cumin, pepper, and coriander. Sprinkle over both sides of the fish. Using your fingertips, gently press the mixture so it adheres to the fish.

In a large nonstick skillet, heat the oil over medium-high heat, swirling to coat the bottom. Place the fish in a single layer in the pan. Reduce the heat to medium. Cook for 4 to 5 minutes on each side, or until the fish flakes easily when tested with a fork. Transfer to a platter. Sprinkle the fish with the remaining 1 tablespoon parsley. Spoon the relish over the fish.

COOK'S TIP Fresh halibut, a good source of omega-3 fatty acids and potassium, may be more widely available in the spring. If you can't find it, try frozen halibut steaks or steaks or fillets from another firm white fish, such as cod or haddock.

RELISH
- ¾ cup chopped mango
- 3 tablespoons golden raisins
- 1 tablespoon finely chopped red bell pepper
- 1 teaspoon snipped fresh Italian (flat-leaf) parsley
- ½ teaspoon white balsamic vinegar

FISH
- 1 teaspoon ground cumin
- ½ teaspoon pepper
- ½ teaspoon ground coriander
- 4 halibut steaks (about 4 ounces each), cut about ¾ inch thick, rinsed and patted dry
- 2 teaspoons olive oil
- 1 tablespoon snipped fresh Italian (flat-leaf) parsley

PER SERVING

calories 193	**cholesterol** 36 mg	**protein** 24 g	**dietary exchanges**
total fat 5.0 g	**sodium** 65 mg	**calcium** 70 mg	1 fruit
saturated 0.5 g	**carbohydrates** 12 g	**potassium** 644 mg	3 lean meat
trans 0.0 g	fiber 1 g		
polyunsaturated 1.0 g	sugars 10 g		
monounsaturated 2.5 g			

HALIBUT
with Cilantro Pesto

Pesto with both Italian and Mexican touches turns simple grilled or broiled fish into a delicious entrée.

SERVES 4 | 3 ounces fish per serving

Lightly spray the grill rack or broiler pan with cooking spray. Preheat the grill on medium high or preheat the broiler.

In a small bowl, stir together the pesto ingredients. Brush half the pesto on one side of the fish. Place the fish with the pesto side up on the grill rack or in the broiler pan. Set the remaining pesto aside.

Grill or broil about 6 inches from the heat for 4 minutes. Turn the fish over. Spread with the remaining pesto. Grill or broil for 4 to 6 minutes, or until the fish flakes easily when tested with a fork (for halibut) or is the desired doneness (for salmon). Watch carefully so the walnuts don't burn.

Cooking spray

PESTO

- ½ cup loosely packed fresh cilantro, coarsely chopped
- 1 medium fresh jalapeño, seeds and ribs discarded, finely chopped (optional)
- 2 tablespoons finely chopped walnuts
- 2 tablespoons shredded or grated Parmesan cheese
- 1 teaspoon grated lime zest
- 1 tablespoon fresh lime juice
- 2 teaspoons olive oil
- 1 medium garlic clove, minced

- 4 halibut or salmon fillets (about 4 ounces each), rinsed and patted dry

PER SERVING

calories 182	**cholesterol** 38 mg	**protein** 25 g	**dietary exchanges**
total fat 8.0 g	**sodium** 105 mg	**calcium** 92 mg	3 very lean meat
saturated 1.5 g	**carbohydrates** 1 g	**potassium** 548 mg	1 fat
trans 0.0 g	fiber 0 g		
polyunsaturated 3.0 g	sugars 0 g		
monounsaturated 3.0 g			

WINE-POACHED SALMON

This fresh salmon dish, which gets its distinctive flavor from a hint of cloves, is so quick and easy that it will become an on-the-go favorite. For a change of taste, try topping the salmon with Yogurt Dill Sauce (page 263).

SERVES 4 | 3 ounces fish per serving

In a large skillet, stir together the water, wine, onion, bay leaf, pepper, cloves, and thyme. Bring to a simmer over medium-high heat. Reduce the heat to medium low and cook, partially covered, for 5 minutes.

Add the fish. If necessary, pour in more water to barely cover. Simmer, covered, for 10 to 15 minutes, or to the desired doneness. Using a slotted spatula or pancake turner, transfer the fish to plates. Discard the liquid, onion, and bay leaf. Serve the fish with the lemon wedges to squeeze over the top.

¾ cup water

¾ cup dry white wine (regular or nonalcoholic)

1 medium onion, chopped

1 medium dried bay leaf

¼ teaspoon pepper

⅛ teaspoon ground cloves

⅛ teaspoon dried thyme, crumbled

1 1-pound salmon fillet (1 to 1½ inches thick), cut into 4 pieces, or 4 salmon steaks (about 4 ounces each), rinsed

1 medium lemon, cut into 4 wedges (optional)

COOK'S TIP ON FRESH SALMON You may prefer salmon fillets to salmon steaks because the fillets have very few, if any, bones. Salmon steaks, cut crosswise through the spine, contain many bones.

PER SERVING

calories 144	**cholesterol** 65 mg	**protein** 25 g	**dietary exchanges**
total fat 4.5 g	**sodium** 83 mg	**calcium** 16 mg	3 lean meat
saturated 0.5 g	**carbohydrates** 0 g	**potassium** 399 mg	
trans 0.0 g	fiber 0 g		
polyunsaturated 1.5 g	sugars 0 g		
monounsaturated 1.0 g			

SALMON, POTATOES, AND GREEN BEANS en Papillote

Wrapping each person's dinner individually in cooking parchment, or en papillote (*en pah-pee-YOHT* or *PAH-peh-loht*), gives the meal a special touch.

SERVES 4 | 3 ounces fish, ½ cup potatoes, and ⅓ cup green beans per serving

Preheat the oven to 425°F. Cut eight 15-inch-long sheets of cooking parchment or aluminum foil. Set aside.

Fill a large saucepan three-fourths full with water. Bring to a boil over high heat. Cook the potatoes for 3 minutes. Add the green beans and cook for 3 minutes, or until the beans are tender-crisp. Drain the potatoes and beans in a colander. Transfer to a large bowl.

Stir in the lemon zest, lemon juice, oil, ⅛ teaspoon pepper, and ⅛ teaspoon salt. Set aside.

Sprinkle the flesh side of the fish with the remaining ⅛ teaspoon pepper and remaining ⅛ teaspoon salt. Using your fingertips, gently press the mixture so it adheres to the fish.

To assemble, slightly mound the potato mixture on the center of four of the sheets of parchment or foil. Place the fish on the potato mixture. Place a lemon slice on each piece of fish. Put one of the remaining four sheets of parchment or foil over each serving. Fold the

- 8 ounces small white or red potatoes, thinly sliced
- 8 ounces green beans, trimmed
- 2 teaspoons grated lemon zest
- 1 tablespoon fresh lemon juice
- 2 teaspoons olive oil
- ⅛ teaspoon pepper and ⅛ teaspoon pepper, divided use
- ⅛ teaspoon salt and ⅛ teaspoon salt, divided use
- 4 salmon fillets with skin (about 5 ounces each), rinsed and patted dry
- 4 lemon slices

edges toward the center. Holding the tops together, fold several times to seal securely. Place the packets on a large baking sheet.

Bake for 10 minutes. Using the tines of a fork, carefully open one packet away from you (to prevent steam burns). If the fish is cooked to the desired doneness, carefully open the remaining packets and serve. If the fish isn't cooked enough, reclose the open packet and continue baking all the packets for about 2 minutes. Serve the fish and vegetables in the packets.

PER SERVING

calories 227	**cholesterol** 65 mg	**protein** 27 g	**dietary exchanges**
total fat 6.5 g	**sodium** 235 mg	**calcium** 47 mg	1 starch
saturated 1.0 g	**carbohydrates** 15 g	**potassium** 764 mg	3 lean meat
trans 0.0 g	fiber 3 g		
polyunsaturated 2.0 g	sugars 1 g		
monounsaturated 3.0 g			

SALMON with Mexican Rub
and Chipotle Sour Cream Sauce

A mildly spicy, citrus-tinged sour cream sauce tops these baked salmon fillets. The ground chipotle adds just a hint of smokiness.

SERVES 4 | 3 ounces fish and 2 tablespoons sauce per serving

Preheat the oven to 350°F. Line a baking sheet with aluminum foil. Lightly spray the foil with cooking spray.

In a small bowl, stir together the Chili Powder, cumin, and salt. Sprinkle over both sides of the fish. Using your fingertips, gently press the rub so it adheres to the fish. Transfer the fish to the baking sheet.

Bake for 20 minutes, or to the desired doneness.

Meanwhile, in a small bowl, stir together the sauce ingredients.

Spoon the sauce over the fish. Squeeze the lemon wedges over all.

Cooking spray
- 1 teaspoon Chili Powder (page 277) or no-salt-added chili powder
- ½ teaspoon ground cumin
- ⅛ teaspoon salt
- 4 salmon fillets (about 4 ounces each), rinsed and patted dry

SAUCE
- ½ cup fat-free sour cream
- 1 tablespoon fresh lime juice
- ¼ teaspoon ground cumin
- ¼ teaspoon ground chipotle or ⅛ to ¼ teaspoon cayenne
- ⅛ teaspoon salt

- 1 medium lemon or lime, cut into 4 wedges

PER SERVING

calories 178	**cholesterol** 70 mg	**protein** 27 g	**dietary exchanges**
total fat 4.5 g	**sodium** 254 mg	**calcium** 83 mg	½ other carbohydrate
saturated 0.5 g	**carbohydrates** 6 g	**potassium** 497 mg	3 lean meat
trans 0.0 g	fiber 0 g		
polyunsaturated 1.5 g	sugars 2 g		
monounsaturated 1.0 g			

GRILLED SALMON FILLET
with Fresh Herbs

Fresh salmon with fresh herbs and lemon—a stellar combination. If you prefer your fish with sauce, this entrée is also great topped with Pineapple-Kiwi Salsa (page 270).

SERVES 4 | 3 ounces fish per serving

Generously spray the grill rack with olive oil spray. Preheat the grill on medium high.

Place the fish with the skin side down on a large plate. Squeeze the juice from one lemon half over the fish. Sprinkle with the dillweed. Using your fingertips, gently press the dillweed so it adheres to the fish.

Thinly slice the remaining lemon half. Lay the slices on the fish. Top with 8 sprigs of thyme.

Grill the fish with the skin side down for 20 minutes, or to the desired doneness. Serve the fish garnished with the remaining 4 sprigs of thyme.

Olive oil spray
- 1 1-pound 4-ounce salmon fillet with skin (tail end preferred), rinsed
- 1 medium lemon, halved crosswise, divided use
- 1½ teaspoons snipped fresh dillweed or ½ teaspoon dried, crumbled
- 12 sprigs of fresh thyme, divided use

PER SERVING

calories 145	**cholesterol** 65 mg	**protein** 25 g	**dietary exchanges**
total fat 4.5 g	**sodium** 83 mg	**calcium** 17 mg	3 lean meat
saturated 0.5 g	**carbohydrates** 1 g	**potassium** 407 mg	
trans 0.0 g	fiber 0 g		
polyunsaturated 1.5 g	sugars 0 g		
monounsaturated 1.0 g			

OREGANO SNAPPER
with Lemon

Sprinkle, bake, and serve—any easier and it wouldn't be called cooking!

SERVES 4 | 3 ounces fish per serving

Preheat the oven to 350°F. Line a baking pan with aluminum foil. Lightly spray with cooking spray.

Place the fish in a single layer in the baking pan.

In a small bowl, stir together the remaining ingredients except the lemon. Sprinkle over the fish. Using your fingertips, gently press the mixture so it adheres to the fish. Lightly spray with cooking spray.

Bake for 10 to 12 minutes, or until the fish flakes easily when tested with a fork. Serve with the lemon wedges to squeeze over the fish.

Cooking spray
- 4 red snapper or other mild white fish fillets (about 4 ounces each), rinsed and patted dry
- 1 teaspoon dried oregano, crumbled
- ½ teaspoon ground cumin
- ¼ teaspoon salt
- ¼ teaspoon pepper

Paprika to taste
- 1 medium lemon, cut into 4 wedges

PER SERVING

calories 114	cholesterol 40 mg	protein 23 g	dietary exchanges
total fat 1.5 g	**sodium** 195 mg	**calcium** 42 mg	3 very lean meat
saturated 0.5 g	**carbohydrates** 1 g	**potassium** 471 mg	
trans 0.0 g	fiber 0 g		
polyunsaturated 0.5 g	sugars 0 g		
monounsaturated 0.5 g			

CAJUN SNAPPER

This intensely flavored entrée is ready in less than 15 minutes. Try it with Zesty Oven-Fried Potatoes (page 250) and stewed okra.

SERVES 4 | 3 ounces fish per serving

In a small bowl, stir together the rub ingredients. Spoon onto one side of each fillet. Using the back of a spoon, spread the rub to cover that side.

In a large skillet, heat the oil over medium-high heat, swirling to coat the bottom. Cook the fish with the coated side down for 4 minutes. Gently turn the fish over and cook for 3 to 4 minutes, or until it flakes easily when tested with a fork. Transfer the fish to plates, leaving any browned bits in the skillet.

Add the water to the skillet, scraping to dislodge the browned bits. Cook for 15 to 20 seconds, or until heated through. Spoon over the fish.

RUB

- 2 teaspoons fresh lemon juice
- 1½ teaspoons Worcestershire sauce (lowest sodium available)
- 1 teaspoon paprika
- ¾ teaspoon chopped fresh thyme or ¼ teaspoon dried, crumbled
- ½ teaspoon red hot-pepper sauce
- ¼ teaspoon garlic powder
- ¼ teaspoon onion powder
- ¼ teaspoon salt

- 4 red snapper or other mild white fish fillets (about 4 ounces each), rinsed and patted dry
- 2 teaspoons olive oil
- 2 tablespoons water

PER SERVING

calories 133	**cholesterol** 40 mg	**protein** 23 g	**dietary exchanges**
total fat 4.0 g	**sodium** 201 mg	**calcium** 39 mg	3 lean meat
saturated 0.5 g	**carbohydrates** 1 g	**potassium** 466 mg	
trans 0.0 g	fiber 0 g		
polyunsaturated 1.0 g	sugars 0 g		
monounsaturated 2.0 g			

SOLE with Vegetables and Dijon Dill Sauce

A citrusy aroma will fill your kitchen as fish fillets and a variety of vegetables bake in foil packets. Spoon on the sauce and enjoy!

SERVES 4 | 3 ounces fish, ½ cup vegetables, and 2 tablespoons sauce per serving

Preheat the oven to 400°F.

In a large nonstick skillet, heat the oil over medium heat, swirling to coat the bottom. Cook the leeks, mushrooms, carrot, and bell pepper for 2 to 3 minutes, or until the carrot slices are tender-crisp, stirring occasionally.

Stir in the sugar snap peas and bouillon granules. Remove from the heat.

Meanwhile, lightly spray four 12-inch square pieces of aluminum foil with cooking spray. Arrange 2 slices of lemon and 2 slices of lime in a single layer in the middle of each piece of foil. Place a fillet on the citrus slices on each piece of foil. Sprinkle with the marjoram and pepper. Using your fingertips, gently press the seasonings so they adhere to the fish. Spoon about ½ cup of the leek mixture onto each fillet. Seal the foil tightly. Transfer the packets with the smooth side down to a baking sheet.

Bake for 20 minutes. Using the tines of a fork, carefully open a packet away from you (to prevent steam burns). If the fish is cooked to the desired doneness, carefully open the remaining packets and serve. If the fish isn't cooked

1 teaspoon olive oil

2 medium leeks (white part only), thinly sliced (about ⅓ cup)

4 ounces medium cremini (brown) or button mushrooms, quartered

1 medium carrot, thinly sliced

½ medium red bell pepper, thinly sliced

1 cup fresh or frozen sugar snap peas, trimmed if fresh

½ teaspoon very low sodium chicken bouillon granules

Cooking spray

1 small lemon, cut into 8 slices and seeded

1 small lime, cut into 8 slices and seeded

4 sole or other mild white fish fillets (about 4 ounces each), rinsed and patted dry

1 teaspoon dried marjoram or dried oregano, crumbled

¼ teaspoon pepper

(continued)

enough, continue baking for about 2 minutes. Transfer the packets to plates.

Meanwhile, in a small bowl, whisk together the sauce ingredients. (The sauce can be made ahead and refrigerated for up to four days.) If desired, heat the sauce in a small saucepan over low heat for 1 to 2 minutes, or until heated through, stirring occasionally. If you prefer, put the sauce in a small microwaveable bowl. Microwave, covered and vented, on 100 percent power (high) for 30 to 45 seconds, stirring once halfway through. Spoon about 2 tablespoons sauce over each serving.

SAUCE

- ½ cup fat-free plain yogurt
- 1 tablespoon Dijon mustard (lowest sodium available)
- 1 teaspoon snipped fresh dillweed or ¼ teaspoon dried, crumbled
- ½ teaspoon grated lemon zest
- 1 teaspoon fresh lemon juice
- ½ teaspoon sugar

PER SERVING

calories 185	**cholesterol** 54 mg	**protein** 24 g	**dietary exchanges**
total fat 3.0 g	**sodium** 206 mg	**calcium** 136 mg	2 vegetable
saturated 0.5 g	**carbohydrates** 16 g	**potassium** 727 mg	½ other carbohydrate
trans 0.0 g	fiber 3 g		3 very lean meat
polyunsaturated 1.0 g	sugars 8 g		
monounsaturated 1.0 g			

HERBED FILLET OF SOLE

Fragrant herbs, tart fresh lemon juice, and a bit of dry mustard flavor these moist broiled sole fillets.

SERVES 4 | 3 ounces fish per serving

Preheat the broiler. Spread the margarine over the bottom of a 13 x 9 x 2-inch broilerproof baking dish. Set aside.

In a small bowl, stir together the remaining ingredients except the fish.

Put the fish in a single layer in the baking dish. Pour half the lemon juice mixture over the fish. Set the remaining mixture aside.

Broil the fish about 4 inches from the heat for 4 minutes with the oven door partially open (to keep the fish from overcooking). Pour the remaining lemon juice mixture over the fish. Broil for 4 to 6 minutes, or until the fish flakes easily when tested with a fork.

2 tablespoons light tub margarine

¼ cup fresh lemon juice

1 tablespoon dried parsley, crumbled

2 teaspoons dried chives, crumbled

½ teaspoon dried tarragon, crumbled

¼ teaspoon dry mustard

4 sole or other mild white fish fillets (about 4 ounces each), rinsed

PER SERVING

calories 98
total fat 1.5 g
  saturated 0.5 g
  trans 0.0 g
  polyunsaturated 0.5 g
  monounsaturated 0.0 g

cholesterol 53 mg
sodium 84 mg
carbohydrates 2 g
  fiber 0 g
  sugars 0 g

protein 19 g
calcium 24 mg
potassium 310 mg

dietary exchanges
3 very lean meat

GARLIC-LIME MARINATED TROUT

A simple citrus marinade is a perfect complement to trout's delicate flavor. Whether you grill or broil the trout, you'll love how easy it is to prepare this dish.

SERVES 4 | 3 ounces fish per serving

In a large shallow dish, stir together the marinade ingredients. Add the fish, turning several times to coat. Cover and refrigerate for 15 minutes to 1 hour.

Lightly spray the grill rack or broiler pan and rack with cooking spray. Preheat the grill on medium high or preheat the broiler.

Transfer the fish with the flesh side up to a large plate, discarding the marinade. Sprinkle the flesh side of the fish with the salt. Using your fingertips, gently press the salt so it adheres to the fish.

If grilling, place the fish with the flesh side down on the grill and grill for 2 to 3 minutes on each side, or until the fish flakes easily when tested with a fork. If broiling, place the fish with the flesh side up on the broiler rack and broil 4 to 5 inches from the heat for 5 to 6 minutes without turning, or until the fish flakes easily when tested with a fork. Serve with the lime wedges to squeeze over the fish.

MARINADE

- 2 teaspoons grated lime zest
- 3 tablespoons fresh lime juice
- 2 teaspoons olive oil
- 1 medium garlic clove, minced
- ⅛ teaspoon pepper

- 4 trout fillets with skin (about 5 ounces each), rinsed
- Cooking spray
- ⅛ teaspoon salt
- 1 medium lime, cut into 4 wedges

PER SERVING

calories 168	**cholesterol** 66 mg	**protein** 24 g	**dietary exchanges**
total fat 7.5 g	**sodium** 132 mg	**calcium** 49 mg	3 lean meat
saturated 1.5 g	**carbohydrates** 0 g	**potassium** 409 mg	
trans 0.0 g	fiber 0 g		
polyunsaturated 1.5 g	sugars 0 g		
monounsaturated 3.5 g			

SAUTÉED TROUT
with Cucumber-Melon Salsa

A summery salsa tops these simply prepared trout fillets. If trout isn't available, serve the salsa with any other sautéed or grilled fish or with shrimp.

SERVES 4 | 3 ounces fish and ½ cup salsa per serving

In a medium bowl, stir together the salsa ingredients. Set aside.

Sprinkle the flesh side of the fish with the cumin, salt, and pepper. Using your fingertips, gently press the mixture so it adheres to the fish.

Put the flour in a medium shallow dish. Add the fish with the flesh side down. Lightly coat that side with the flour, shaking off any excess.

In a large nonstick skillet, heat 2 teaspoons oil over medium-high heat, swirling to coat the bottom. Cook 2 pieces of the fish with the flesh side down for 2 minutes, or until browned. Turn over and cook for 2 minutes, or until the fish flakes easily when tested with a fork. Transfer to a large plate. Cover to keep warm.

Put the remaining 1 teaspoon oil in the skillet, swirling to coat the bottom. Cook the remaining 2 pieces of fish. Transfer all the fish to plates. Top with the salsa. Serve with the lemon wedges to squeeze over all.

SALSA
- 1 cup diced cantaloupe
- 1 cup diced seeded cucumber (English, or hothouse, preferred)
- 1 tablespoon snipped fresh mint
- ½ teaspoon grated lemon zest
- 2 teaspoons fresh lemon juice
- 1 teaspoon seeded and minced fresh jalapeño
- ⅛ teaspoon ground cumin

- 4 trout fillets with skin (about 5 ounces each), rinsed and patted dry
- ½ teaspoon ground cumin
- ⅛ teaspoon salt
- ⅛ teaspoon pepper
- 2 tablespoons flour
- 2 teaspoons canola or corn oil and 1 teaspoon canola or corn oil, divided use
- 1 medium lemon, cut into 4 wedges

PER SERVING

calories 234	**cholesterol** 66 mg	**protein** 25 g	**dietary exchanges**
total fat 11.0 g	**sodium** 140 mg	**calcium** 64 mg	½ fruit
saturated 1.5 g	**carbohydrates** 8 g	**potassium** 569 mg	3 lean meat
trans 0.0 g	fiber 1 g		½ fat
polyunsaturated 2.5 g	sugars 4 g		
monounsaturated 6.0 g			

GRILLED TUNA STEAKS
with Thyme

You'll have time to do some stretches, go for a walk, and even begin to make a green salad while the tuna absorbs the flavors of an herby lemon juice mixture.

SERVES 4 | 3 ounces fish per serving

In a small bowl, stir together the lemon juice, parsley, oil, thyme, and pepper.

Put the fish in a single layer in a large glass baking dish. Rub the fish on both sides with the lemon juice mixture. Cover and refrigerate for 30 minutes to 1 hour.

Lightly spray the grill rack with cooking spray. Preheat the grill on medium high.

Grill the tuna for 3 to 5 minutes on each side, or to the desired doneness.

2 tablespoons fresh lemon juice

1 tablespoon dried parsley, crumbled

2 teaspoons olive oil

1 teaspoon dried thyme, crumbled

½ teaspoon pepper

4 tuna steaks (about 4 ounces each), rinsed

Cooking spray

COOK'S TIP ON GRILLING FISH For an attractive crosshatch pattern, grill the fish on one side for about one-quarter of the total grilling time. Keeping the same side down, rotate the fish 90 degrees. Grill for about one-quarter of the total grilling time. Turn the fish over and repeat.

PER SERVING

calories 147	**cholesterol** 51 mg	**protein** 27 g	**dietary exchanges**
total fat 3.5 g	**sodium** 44 mg	**calcium** 28 mg	3 very lean meat
saturated 0.5 g	**carbohydrates** 1 g	**potassium** 533 mg	
trans 0.0 g	fiber 0 g		
polyunsaturated 0.5 g	sugars 0 g		
monounsaturated 2.0 g			

SMOKED-PAPRIKA TUNA STEAKS with Spinach

Garlic-enhanced wilted spinach is the perfect accompaniment for tuna steaks seasoned with smoked paprika and oregano.

SERVES 4 | 3 ounces fish and ½ cup spinach per serving

In a small bowl, whisk together the orange juice, wine, and 1 teaspoon oil.

Put the fish in a glass casserole dish large enough to hold the steaks in a single layer. Pour in the orange juice mixture. Turn to coat. Cover and refrigerate for 30 minutes.

Meanwhile, preheat the oven to 450°F. Lightly spray a medium baking sheet with cooking spray.

In a small bowl, stir together the brown sugar, paprika, and oregano.

Transfer the fish to the baking sheet, discarding any remaining marinade. Sprinkle the brown sugar mixture over the top side of the fish. Using your fingertips, gently press the mixture so it adheres to the fish.

Bake with the seasoned side up for 7 to 10 minutes, or until the desired doneness.

2 tablespoons fresh orange juice

2 tablespoons dry white wine (regular or nonalcoholic)

1 teaspoon olive oil and 1 teaspoon olive oil, divided use

1 1-pound tuna steak (about 1 inch thick), rinsed, cut into 4 pieces

Cooking spray

1 tablespoon firmly packed light brown sugar

1 tablespoon smoked paprika

2 teaspoons ground oregano, crumbled

12 ounces baby spinach (about 12 cups)

2 medium garlic cloves, minced

Meanwhile, in a large nonstick skillet, heat the remaining 1 teaspoon oil over medium-high heat, swirling to coat the bottom. Cook the spinach and garlic for 2 minutes, or until the spinach is wilted, stirring frequently. Spoon about ½ cup spinach onto each plate, spreading to make beds for the fish. Serve the fish on the spinach.

PER SERVING

calories 187	**cholesterol** 53 mg	**protein** 28 g	**dietary exchanges**
total fat 4.0 g	**sodium** 112 mg	**calcium** 141 mg	½ other carbohydrate
saturated 1.0 g	**carbohydrates** 9 g	**potassium** 1,020 mg	3 lean meat
trans 0.0 g	fiber 3 g		
polyunsaturated 1.0 g	sugars 5 g		
monounsaturated 2.0 g			

TUNA PENNE CASSEROLE

Curry powder provides a Middle Eastern twist for homey tuna casserole. Using cornstarch and milk instead of a canned cream soup really cuts the sodium in this comfort-food dish.

SERVES 4 | 1 cup per serving

Prepare the pasta using the package directions, omitting the salt. Drain well in a colander. Set aside.

Meanwhile, lightly spray a large broilerproof skillet with cooking spray. Add the oil, swirling to coat the bottom. Cook the onion over medium-high heat for 3 minutes, or until soft, stirring frequently. Set aside.

Preheat the broiler if using the topping.

Put the cornstarch in a cup. Add the water, whisking to dissolve. Set aside.

Whisk the milk, parsley, curry powder, salt, onion powder, and pepper into the onion. Cook, still over medium-high heat, for 5 minutes, or until the milk mixture is hot.

Gently whisk in the cornstarch mixture. Continue to gently whisk for 3 to 5 minutes, or until slightly thickened. Remove from the heat.

1½ cups dried whole-grain penne or macaroni

Cooking spray

1 teaspoon canola or corn oil

¼ cup chopped onion

1 tablespoon cornstarch

3 tablespoons water

1½ cups fat-free milk

1 tablespoon finely snipped fresh parsley or 1 teaspoon dried, crumbled

1 teaspoon curry powder

¼ teaspoon salt

¼ teaspoon onion powder

⅛ teaspoon pepper

1 cup canned no-salt-added French-style green beans, drained

¾ cup drained no-salt-added canned diced tomatoes

1 5-ounce can very low sodium albacore tuna, packed in water, drained and flaked

(continued)

Stir in the beans, tomatoes, tuna, and pasta.

In a small bowl, stir together the panko and margarine. Sprinkle over the casserole.

Broil about 4 inches from the heat for 30 seconds to 1 minute, or until the topping is browned.

TOPPING (OPTIONAL)

¼ cup plus 2 tablespoons panko (Japanese bread crumbs)

1 tablespoon light tub margarine, melted

COOK'S TIP ON CORNSTARCH Cornstarch needs gentle treatment. Too much heat or stirring will cause a cornstarch-thickened sauce to become thin.

PER SERVING

calories 254	cholesterol 17 mg	protein 18 g	dietary exchanges
total fat 3.0 g	sodium 212 mg	calcium 162 mg	2½ starch
saturated 0.5 g	carbohydrates 41 g	potassium 482 mg	1 vegetable
trans 0.0 g	fiber 5 g		1½ very lean meat
polyunsaturated 1.0 g	sugars 6 g		
monounsaturated 1.0 g			

PER SERVING
WITH OPTIONAL INGREDIENTS

calories 279	cholesterol 17 mg	protein 18 g	dietary exchanges
total fat 4.0 g	sodium 241 mg	calcium 162 mg	2½ starch
saturated 0.5 g	carbohydrates 44 g	potassium 484 mg	1 vegetable
trans 0.0 g	fiber 5 g		1½ very lean meat
polyunsaturated 1.0 g	sugars 6 g		
monounsaturated 2.0 g			

TUNA TERIYAKI STIR-FRY

Stir-fry fresh albacore tuna, plump sugar snap peas, and thin slices of green onions, carrot, and red bell pepper, then serve over brown rice.

SERVES 4 | 1 cup tuna and vegetable mixture and ½ cup rice per serving

Prepare the rice using the package directions, omitting the salt and margarine. Cover to keep warm. Set aside.

Meanwhile, in a small bowl, whisk together the glaze ingredients. Set aside.

In a large nonstick skillet, heat the oil over medium-high heat, swirling to coat the bottom. Cook the fish, garlic, and gingerroot for 3 to 4 minutes, or until the fish is golden brown on all sides (it will still be slightly pink inside), stirring constantly.

Stir in the sugar snap peas, green onions, carrot, and bell pepper. Cook for 2 to 3 minutes, or until the vegetables are tender-crisp, stirring constantly.

Make a well in the center of the fish and vegetables. Pour in the glaze mixture. Simmer for 1 to 2 minutes, or until the glaze is thickened, stirring occasionally in the well only. Stir the fish and vegetables into the thickened glaze. Cook for 1 minute, or until the mixture is heated through, stirring constantly. Serve over the rice.

1 cup uncooked instant brown rice

GLAZE
¼ cup water

2 tablespoons teriyaki sauce (lowest sodium available)

½ teaspoon cornstarch

½ teaspoon toasted sesame oil

---

1 teaspoon canola or corn oil

4 tuna steaks (about 4 ounces each), rinsed and patted dry, cut into ¾-inch cubes

2 medium garlic cloves, minced

1 teaspoon grated peeled gingerroot

4 ounces sugar snap peas, trimmed

4 medium green onions, thinly sliced

1 medium carrot, thinly sliced

½ medium red bell pepper, thinly sliced

PER SERVING

calories 343	**cholesterol** 43 mg	**protein** 32 g	**dietary exchanges**
total fat 11.0 g	**sodium** 301 mg	**calcium** 50 mg	1½ starch
saturated 2.5 g	**carbohydrates** 27 g	**potassium** 726 mg	1 vegetable
trans 0.0 g	fiber 4 g		3 lean meat
polyunsaturated 1.0 g	sugars 5 g		
monounsaturated 1.5 g			

SHRIMP AND SPINACH PASTA

You won't need a separate pan to cook the spinach for this attractive dish. Just pour the pasta and cooking water over the spinach to blanch it. Quick and easy!

SERVES 4 | 1½ cups per serving

Prepare the pasta using the package directions, omitting the salt.

Put the spinach in a large colander in the sink. Pour the pasta and cooking water over the spinach. Drain well.

Meanwhile, in a large nonstick skillet, heat the oil over medium-high heat, swirling to coat the bottom. Cook the onion and bell pepper for about 3 minutes, or until soft, stirring frequently.

Stir in the shrimp and garlic. Cook for 3 minutes, or until the shrimp are pink, stirring frequently.

Add the pasta mixture, pepper, and salt to the shrimp mixture, stirring to combine. Remove from the heat. Stir in the lemon zest and lemon juice.

8 ounces dried whole-grain linguine, spaghetti, or vermicelli

6 ounces spinach, chopped (about 4 cups)

2 teaspoons olive oil

1 small red onion, thinly sliced crosswise

1 small red bell pepper, cut into thin strips

1 pound raw medium shrimp, peeled, rinsed, and patted dry

2 medium garlic cloves, minced

¼ teaspoon pepper

⅛ teaspoon salt

2 teaspoons grated lemon zest

3 tablespoons fresh lemon juice

PER SERVING

calories 331	**cholesterol** 168 mg	**protein** 28 g	**dietary exchanges**
total fat 4.0 g	**sodium** 306 mg	**calcium** 109 mg	3 starch
saturated 0.5 g	**carbohydrates** 49 g	**potassium** 604 mg	1 vegetable
trans 0.0 g	fiber 9 g		3 very lean meat
polyunsaturated 1.0 g	sugars 4 g		
monounsaturated 2.0 g			

RISOTTO
with Shrimp and Vegetables

The delicate crunch of snow peas and the burst of flavor from lemon zest add interesting surprises to this creamy dish.

SERVES 5 | 1 cup per serving

In a medium saucepan, heat the oil over medium heat, swirling to coat the bottom. Cook the onion, bell pepper, and garlic for 2 to 3 minutes, or until tender-crisp, stirring frequently.

Stir in the rice. Cook for 5 minutes, stirring frequently.

Add 1½ cups broth and the pepper. Increase the heat to high and bring to a boil, stirring occasionally. Reduce the heat and simmer for 5 minutes, stirring occasionally. The rice will be slightly plump, the liquid will not be entirely absorbed, and the mixture will have a thick, soupy or stewlike consistency.

Stir in the wine and remaining ½ cup broth. Increase the heat to high and bring to a simmer. Reduce the heat to medium high and cook for 8 to 10 minutes, stirring constantly (a small amount of liquid should remain).

1 teaspoon olive oil
½ medium onion, sliced
½ medium red bell pepper, chopped
2 medium garlic cloves, minced
1 cup uncooked arborio rice
1½ cups and ½ cup Chicken Broth (page 50) or commercial fat-free, low-sodium chicken broth, divided use
⅛ teaspoon pepper
1 cup dry white wine (regular or nonalcoholic)
1 pound raw large shrimp, peeled, rinsed, and patted dry
6 ounces snow peas, trimmed and halved crosswise (about 2 cups)
½ cup water

(continued)

Stir in the shrimp, snow peas, and water. Reduce the heat to medium and cook for 2 to 3 minutes, or until the liquid is almost absorbed, stirring constantly. The rice should be just tender and slightly creamy, and the shrimp should be pink.

Stir in the remaining ingredients.

3 tablespoons shredded or grated Romano cheese

1 tablespoon snipped fresh dillweed

1 tablespoon thinly sliced green onions (green part only)

Zest of 1 small lemon cut into very thin strips

COOK'S TIP If the liquid is absorbed before the rice reaches the just-tender stage, gradually add more broth, wine, or water. Arborio rice is usually used in risottos, but you can substitute a medium-grain rice if you prefer. It won't be quite as creamy, however.

PER SERVING

calories 265	**cholesterol** 136 mg	**protein** 20 g	**dietary exchanges**
total fat 2.0 g	**sodium** 192 mg	**calcium** 70 mg	2 starch
saturated 0.5 g	**carbohydrates** 34 g	**potassium** 327 mg	1 vegetable
trans 0.0 g	fiber 2 g		2 very lean meat
polyunsaturated 0.5 g	sugars 3 g		
monounsaturated 1.0 g			

SCALLOPS AND BOK CHOY
with Balsamic Sauce

On their own, scallops have a rich, sweet flavor. When topped with this bold balsamic sauce, they're transformed into an extraordinary dish. Serve the scallops and vegetables over steamed rice and add a tossed salad with Sesame-Ginger Dressing (page 95) for a delectable dinner.

SERVES 4 | 3 ounces scallops per serving

In a large nonstick skillet, heat the oil over medium-high heat, swirling to coat the bottom. Cook the scallops in a single layer with some space between the pieces (so they don't steam). Cook for 1 minute, stirring occasionally after 30 seconds. (If the scallops were frozen, they may need to cook for an additional 1 to 2 minutes to evaporate the extra liquid they release.)

Stir in the remaining ingredients except the vinegar. Cook, covered, for 1 to 2 minutes, or until the scallops are cooked through (white and opaque, not translucent, in the center), stirring occasionally. Watch carefully; scallops become rubbery when overcooked by even 1 or 2 minutes. Using a slotted spoon, transfer the scallop mixture to a serving platter. Cover to keep warm.

Add the vinegar to the liquid in the skillet. Cook for 1 to 2 minutes, or until the liquid is reduced by half. Pour over the scallops.

1 teaspoon olive oil

1 pound bay scallops, rinsed and patted dry

4 stalks of bok choy, ends trimmed, stalks and leaves cut crosswise into ½-inch slices

½ cup roasted red bell peppers, cut into thin strips

2 medium green onions, cut into 1-inch pieces

¼ cup Chicken Broth (page 50) or commercial fat-free, low-sodium chicken broth

2 medium garlic cloves, minced

⅛ teaspoon pepper

2 tablespoons balsamic vinegar

COOK'S TIP ON SCALLOPS When scallops are called for, you can use either sea or bay scallops. Bay scallops (as many as 40 per pound) are milder—and more expensive—than sea scallops (12 to 15 per pound). To substitute sea scallops for bay, cut the sea scallops in halves, quarters, or slices.

COOK'S TIP ON BOK CHOY Look for bok choy, with its long white stalks and large dark green leaves, near the cabbage in the produce section. Slices of raw bok choy stalks add a pleasant crunch to salads. Both the stalks and the leaves are good in stir-fry dishes and soups.

PER SERVING

calories 128	**cholesterol** 37 mg	**protein** 20 g	**dietary exchanges**
total fat 2.0 g	**sodium** 213 mg	**calcium** 47 mg	½ other carbohydrate
saturated 0.5 g	**carbohydrates** 7 g	**potassium** 474 mg	3 very lean meat
trans 0.0 g	fiber 1 g		
polyunsaturated 0.5 g	sugars 2 g		
monounsaturated 1.0 g			

SPANISH-STYLE CRAB AND VEGETABLE TORTILLA

In Mexico, a tortilla is a type of unleavened bread, but in Spain, a tortilla is an omelet, often served open-face.

SERVES 4 | 1 wedge per serving

Lightly spray a medium skillet with olive oil spray. Cook the vegetables over medium-low heat for 3 minutes, stirring occasionally.

Stir in the remaining ingredients. Cook for 1 minute, scrambling lightly and constantly with a fork. Cook, covered, for 11 to 14 minutes, or until the center of the tortilla is firm and doesn't run. Cut the tortilla into 4 wedges.

Olive oil spray

1 cup frozen vegetables, such as artichoke hearts, asparagus, green peas and carrots, or mixed vegetables (4 to 5 ounces), cut into bite-size pieces if needed

1½ cups egg substitute

4 ounces fresh, frozen, or canned crab (about ¾ cup), all cartilage and shell discarded, thawed if frozen, drained if canned

¾ teaspoon finely snipped fresh dillweed or ¼ teaspoon dried, crumbled

Pepper to taste

PER SERVING

calories 95	**cholesterol** 22 mg	**protein** 17 g	**dietary exchanges**
total fat 0.5 g	**sodium** 317 mg	**calcium** 57 mg	1 vegetable
saturated 0.0 g	**carbohydrates** 6 g	**potassium** 356 mg	2 very lean meat
trans 0.0 g	fiber 2 g		
polyunsaturated 0.0 g	sugars 2 g		
monounsaturated 0.0 g			

POULTRY

CHICKEN DIJON

A smooth Dijon sauce enhances the combination of chicken and colorful vegetables. Try this dish with whole-wheat couscous and melon slices.

SERVES 6 | 3 ounces chicken and ⅓ cup vegetables per serving

Sprinkle both sides of the chicken with the pepper. Using your fingertips, gently press the pepper so it adheres to the chicken.

In a large nonstick skillet, heat the oil over medium-high heat, swirling to coat the bottom. Cook the chicken for 2 minutes on each side (the chicken won't be done at this point).

Stir in the broth, carrots, zucchini, bell pepper, and garlic. Cook, covered, for 5 to 8 minutes, or until the chicken is no longer pink in the center and the vegetables are tender, stirring occasionally. Using a slotted spoon, transfer the chicken and vegetables to a plate. Leave the liquid in the skillet. Cover the plate to keep warm.

In a small bowl, whisk together the milk and flour. Add with the margarine and mustard to the liquid in the skillet. Bring to a simmer over medium-high heat, whisking occasionally. Cook for 2 to 3 minutes, or until thickened, whisking occasionally. Pour over the chicken and vegetables. Sprinkle with the parsley.

6 boneless, skinless chicken breast halves (about 4 ounces each), all visible fat discarded, flattened to ½-inch thickness

¼ teaspoon pepper

2 teaspoons olive oil

½ cup Chicken Broth (page 50) or commercial fat-free, low-sodium chicken broth

2 medium carrots, sliced

1 medium zucchini, sliced

½ medium red bell pepper, cut into strips

1 medium garlic clove, minced

½ cup fat-free milk

2 tablespoons all-purpose flour

2 tablespoons light tub margarine

1 to 2 teaspoons Dijon mustard (lowest sodium available)

1 tablespoon snipped fresh parsley or 1 teaspoon dried, crumbled

PER SERVING

calories 190	**cholesterol** 66 mg	**protein** 28 g	**dietary exchanges**
total fat 4.5 g	**sodium** 161 mg	**calcium** 55 mg	½ other carbohydrate
saturated 0.5 g	**carbohydrates** 8 g	**potassium** 527 mg	3 lean meat
trans 0.0 g	fiber 1 g		
polyunsaturated 1.0 g	sugars 3 g		
monounsaturated 2.5 g			

SEARED CHICKEN
with Fresh Pineapple, Ginger, and Mint Salsa

For a refreshing break from the usual vegetable salsa, toss together an aromatic blend of fresh pineapple, grated ginger, mint, and a splash of fresh lemon.

SERVES 4 | 3 ounces chicken and ¼ cup salsa per serving

In a small bowl, stir together the salsa ingredients. Set aside.

In another small bowl, stir together the Chili Powder, thyme, allspice, pepper, and salt. Sprinkle over both sides of the chicken. Using your fingertips, gently press the mixture so it adheres to the chicken.

Lightly spray a large skillet with cooking spray. Heat over medium-high heat. Cook the chicken for 4 minutes. Turn the chicken over and lightly spray with cooking spray. Cook for 2 to 4 minutes, or until no longer pink in the center. Serve the chicken with the salsa on the side.

SALSA

- 1 cup finely chopped fresh pineapple
- 3 tablespoons chopped fresh mint or snipped fresh cilantro
- 2 tablespoons finely chopped red onion
- 1 tablespoon fresh lemon juice
- ¾ teaspoon grated peeled gingerroot

- 1 teaspoon Chili Powder (page 277) or no-salt-added chili powder
- ½ teaspoon dried thyme, crumbled
- ¼ teaspoon ground allspice
- ¼ teaspoon pepper
- ¼ teaspoon salt
- 4 boneless, skinless chicken breast halves (about 4 ounces each), all visible fat discarded

Cooking spray

PER SERVING

calories 154	**cholesterol** 66 mg	**protein** 27 g	**dietary exchanges**
total fat 1.5 g	**sodium** 222 mg	**calcium** 35 mg	½ fruit
saturated 0.5 g	**carbohydrates** 7 g	**potassium** 366 mg	3 very lean meat
trans 0.0 g	fiber 1 g		
polyunsaturated 0.5 g	sugars 4 g		
monounsaturated 0.5 g			

GLAZED RASPBERRY-GINGER CHICKEN

A showpiece, this incredibly easy and elegant entrée pairs chicken glazed with a peppery raspberry mixture and steamed sweet potatoes seasoned with sugar and cinnamon.

SERVES 4 | 3 ounces chicken and ¾ cup sweet potatoes per serving

In a small bowl, whisk together the glaze ingredients. Set aside.

Lightly spray a large skillet with cooking spray. Heat over medium-high heat. Put the chicken in the skillet and reduce the heat to medium. Cook for 4 minutes. Turn the chicken over. Top each piece with 1 tablespoon glaze, reserving the remaining glaze. Cook for 2 to 4 minutes, or until the chicken is no longer pink in the center. Transfer to a large plate.

Meanwhile, in a large saucepan, steam the potato slices for 10 to 12 minutes, or until tender. Drain well. Arrange on a serving plate, leaving space for the chicken in the center. Cover to keep warm.

Add the remaining glaze to the skillet. Bring to a boil over high heat. Boil for 2 minutes, or until the mixture begins to thicken slightly, scraping the skillet frequently.

GLAZE

½ cup all-fruit seedless raspberry spread

2 to 3 tablespoons cider vinegar

1 teaspoon grated peeled gingerroot or ¼ teaspoon ground ginger

¼ teaspoon salt

⅛ to ¼ teaspoon crushed red pepper flakes

Cooking spray

4 boneless, skinless chicken breast halves (about 4 ounces each), all visible fat discarded

1 pound sweet potatoes, peeled and cut crosswise into ½-inch slices

2 teaspoons sugar

⅛ teaspoon ground cinnamon

Return the chicken to the skillet and cook for about 2 minutes, or until richly glazed and beginning to darken intensely, turning constantly. Transfer the chicken to the center of the plate with the potatoes.

In another small bowl, stir together the sugar and cinnamon. Sprinkle over the potatoes.

PER SERVING

calories 303	cholesterol 66 mg	protein 28 g	dietary exchanges
total fat 1.5 g	sodium 281 mg	calcium 32 mg	1½ starch
saturated 0.5 g	carbohydrates 42 g	potassium 683 mg	1½ other carbohydrate
trans 0.0 g	fiber 4 g		3 very lean meat
polyunsaturated 0.5 g	sugars 24 g		
monounsaturated 0.5 g			

CURRIED CHICKEN KEBABS
with Yogurt Dipping Sauce

The yogurt dipping sauce, full of fresh basil and a hint of curry, makes this dish especially fragrant and flavorful. Try it with a side of quinoa.

SERVES 4 | 3 ounces chicken, heaping ⅔ cup grilled vegetables, and 1½ tablespoons dipping sauce per serving

In a food processor or blender, process the yogurt, basil, and 1 wedge of onion until smooth. Pour the mixture into a medium bowl. Set the remaining onion wedges aside.

Stir the curry powder and pepper into the yogurt mixture. Transfer ⅓ cup of the mixture to a small bowl. Cover and refrigerate to serve as the dipping sauce.

Add the chicken to the remaining yogurt mixture, stirring to coat. Cover and refrigerate for 30 minutes to 4 hours.

Meanwhile, if using wooden skewers, soak seven 10-inch skewers for at least 10 minutes in cold water to keep them from charring or use metal skewers, lightly spraying with cooking spray.

Lightly spray the grill rack with cooking spray. Preheat the grill on medium high.

6 ounces fat-free plain yogurt

1 cup packed fresh basil (about 2½ ounces)

1 medium red onion, cut into 3 wedges, each wedge cut into 3 wedges (9 wedges total), divided use

½ teaspoon curry powder

¼ teaspoon pepper

1 pound boneless, skinless chicken breast halves, all visible fat discarded, cut into 1-inch cubes

Cooking spray

1 medium zucchini, halved lengthwise, each half cut crosswise into 8 pieces

1 medium green bell pepper, cut into 16 squares

16 cherry tomatoes

Thread the chicken onto 3 skewers, discarding the marinade. Use one of the remaining 4 skewers for each of the vegetables—zucchini, bell pepper, tomatoes, and remaining 8 onion wedges. Lightly spray the kebabs with cooking spray.

Arrange the kebabs in a single layer on the grill. Cook, covered, for 12 to 14 minutes, or until the chicken is no longer pink in the center and the vegetables are tender, turning occasionally to cook evenly. Transfer the kebabs to a rimmed baking sheet as they become ready.

Slide the chicken and vegetables from the skewers onto a platter. Serve with the reserved ⅓ cup dipping sauce.

PER SERVING

calories 189	**cholesterol** 67 mg	**protein** 31 g	**dietary exchanges**
total fat 2.0 g	**sodium** 119 mg	**calcium** 137 mg	2 vegetable
saturated 0.5 g	**carbohydrates** 12 g	**potassium** 780 mg	3 very lean meat
trans 0.0 g	fiber 2 g		
polyunsaturated 0.5 g	sugars 8 g		
monounsaturated 0.5 g			

BAKED CHICKEN, TOMATO, AND ZUCCHINI PACKETS

When you're rushed for dinner, try this all-in-one-packet combo of chicken and fresh vegetables. While the packets bake, boil some whole-grain pasta to serve on the side.

SERVES 4 | 3 ounces chicken and ⅔ cup vegetables per serving

Preheat the oven to 425°F. Cut eight 15-inch-long sheets of cooking parchment or aluminum foil. Set aside.

In a large bowl, combine the tomatoes, zucchini, onion, oil, 1 teaspoon lime zest, the lime juice, ¼ teaspoon cumin, and ⅛ teaspoon salt, stirring to coat. Set aside.

In a small bowl, stir together the remaining 2 teaspoons lime zest, remaining ¼ teaspoon cumin, and remaining ⅛ teaspoon salt. Sprinkle on both sides of the chicken. Using your finger-tips, gently press the mixture so it adheres to the chicken.

Slightly mound the tomato mixture on the center of four of the parchment or foil sheets. Place the chicken on the tomato mixture. Place the remaining four sheets of parchment or foil over the chicken. Fold the edges toward the center. Holding the tops together, fold several times to seal securely. Place the packets on a large baking sheet.

1½ cups cherry tomatoes, halved

1 medium zucchini, quartered lengthwise and thinly sliced crosswise

¼ cup thinly sliced red onion

2 teaspoons olive oil

1 teaspoon grated lime zest and 2 teaspoons grated lime zest, divided use

1 tablespoon fresh lime juice

¼ teaspoon ground cumin and ¼ teaspoon ground cumin, divided use

⅛ teaspoon salt and ⅛ teaspoon salt, divided use

4 boneless, skinless chicken breast halves (about 4 ounces each), all visible fat discarded

Bake for 20 minutes. Using the tines of a fork, carefully open a packet away from you (to prevent steam burns). If the chicken is no longer pink in the center, carefully open the remaining packets and serve. If the chicken isn't done, reclose the open packet and continue baking all the packets for about 5 minutes. Serve the chicken and vegetables in the packets.

PER SERVING

calories 176	**cholesterol** 66 mg	**protein** 28 g	**dietary exchanges**
total fat 4.0 g	**sodium** 233 mg	**calcium** 30 mg	1 vegetable
saturated 0.5 g	**carbohydrates** 7 g	**potassium** 629 mg	3 lean meat
trans 0.0 g	fiber 2 g		
polyunsaturated 0.5 g	sugars 4 g		
monounsaturated 2.0 g			

BLUE CHEESE AND BASIL CHICKEN

Just a little full-flavored blue cheese is enough to give a kick to this very-simple-to-fix entrée.

SERVES 4 | 3 ounces chicken per serving

Sprinkle the basil, pepper, and salt over both sides of the chicken. Using your fingertips, gently press the seasonings so they adhere to the chicken.

Lightly spray a large skillet with cooking spray. Heat over medium-high heat. Cook the chicken for 4 minutes. Turn over and cook for 2 to 4 minutes, or until no longer pink in the center. Remove the skillet from the heat.

Sprinkle the chicken with the blue cheese and green onion. Let stand, covered, for 2 to 3 minutes, or until the cheese is slightly melted.

1 teaspoon dried basil, crumbled

¼ teaspoon pepper

⅛ teaspoon salt

4 boneless, skinless chicken breast halves (about 4 ounces each), all visible fat discarded

Cooking spray

¼ cup crumbled blue cheese

1 medium green onion, finely chopped

PER SERVING

calories 154
total fat 3.5 g
  saturated 1.5 g
  trans 0.0 g
  polyunsaturated 0.5 g
  monounsaturated 1.0 g

cholesterol 71 mg
sodium 247 mg
carbohydrates 1 g
  fiber 0 g
  sugars 0 g

protein 28 g
calcium 58 mg
potassium 339 mg

dietary exchanges
3 lean meat

CHICKEN MARENGO

This dish stars chicken that is seared, then cooked in an herbed tomato and wine sauce to keep it moist and tender. Serve on a bed of spinach pasta and add a tossed salad for a tempting and nutritious meal.

SERVES 6 | 3 ounces chicken and ½ cup vegetables and sauce per serving

Sprinkle the pepper over both sides of the chicken. Using your fingertips, gently press the pepper so it adheres to the chicken.

In a large nonstick skillet, heat the oil over medium-high heat, swirling to coat the bottom. Cook the chicken for 3 minutes on each side (the chicken won't be done at this point). Transfer to a plate. Set aside.

In the same skillet, stir together the mushrooms, onion, and garlic. Cook over medium heat for 3 to 4 minutes, or until soft, stirring occasionally.

Stir in the remaining ingredients. Return the chicken to the skillet. Spoon the sauce over the chicken. Increase the heat to medium high and bring to a simmer. Reduce the heat to medium low. Cook, covered, for 25 minutes.

½ teaspoon pepper

6 boneless, skinless chicken breast halves (about 4 ounces each), all visible fat discarded

2 teaspoons olive oil

8 ounces button mushrooms, sliced

1 medium red onion, chopped

2 medium garlic cloves, minced

1 14.5-ounce can diced no-salt-added tomatoes, undrained

½ cup marsala or dry white wine (regular or nonalcoholic)

1 teaspoon sugar

1 teaspoon dried oregano, crumbled

½ teaspoon dried thyme, crumbled

¼ to ½ teaspoon crushed red pepper flakes (optional)

PER SERVING

calories 203	**cholesterol** 66 mg	**protein** 28 g	**dietary exchanges**
total fat 3.0 g	**sodium** 85 mg	**calcium** 50 mg	½ other carbohydrate
saturated 0.5 g	**carbohydrates** 10 g	**potassium** 599 mg	3 very lean meat
trans 0.0 g	fiber 2 g		
polyunsaturated 0.5 g	sugars 6 g		
monounsaturated 1.5 g			

BLACKENED CHICKEN
with Mustard Aïoli

Aïoli (*ay-OH-lee*), a mixture of garlic and mayonnaise, lends itself to a variety of interpretations. Here it gets a slightly sweet, slightly tangy lift from tarragon and Dijon mustard.

SERVES 4 | 3 ounces chicken and 2 tablespoons aïoli per serving

Sprinkle the seasoning blend over both sides of the chicken. Using your fingertips, gently press the seasoning blend so it adheres to the chicken.

Lightly spray a large skillet with cooking spray. Heat over medium-high heat. Cook the chicken for 4 minutes. Turn the chicken over. Lightly spray the chicken with cooking spray. Cook for 2 to 4 minutes, or until no longer pink in the center.

Meanwhile, in a small bowl, stir together the aïoli ingredients. Serve with the chicken.

1 teaspoon Creole Seasoning (page 278) or salt-free Creole or Cajun seasoning blend

4 boneless, skinless chicken breast halves (about 4 ounces each), all visible fat discarded

Cooking spray

AÏOLI

¼ cup plus 2 table-spoons fat-free sour cream

2 tablespoons light mayonnaise

2 teaspoons Dijon mustard (lowest sodium available)

1½ teaspoons snipped fresh tarragon or ½ teaspoon dried, crumbled

½ medium garlic clove, minced

⅛ teaspoon salt

⅛ teaspoon red hot-pepper sauce

PER SERVING

calories 171	**cholesterol** 72 mg	**protein** 28 g	**dietary exchanges**
total fat 3.5 g	**sodium** 283 mg	**calcium** 65 mg	½ other carbohydrate
saturated 0.5 g	**carbohydrates** 5 g	**potassium** 361 mg	3 very lean meat
trans 0.0 g	fiber 0 g		
polyunsaturated 1.5 g	sugars 2 g		
monounsaturated 0.5 g			

CHICKEN
with Yogurt-Cilantro Sauce

This dish is so scrumptious that even low-salt skeptics will be clamoring for a sample. You won't have to spend much time in the kitchen, but remember to allow time for marinating.

SERVES 4 | 3 ounces chicken and 2 tablespoons sauce per serving

In a large glass dish, stir together the lime juice, oil, and pepper. Add the chicken, turning to coat. Cover and refrigerate for 30 minutes to 8 hours, turning occasionally. Remove the chicken from the refrigerator 5 to 10 minutes before cooking.

In a small bowl, stir together the yogurt, cilantro, mint, and cumin. Set aside.

Lightly spray the broiler pan and rack or the grill rack with cooking spray. Preheat the broiler or preheat the grill on medium high.

Broil the chicken 4 to 5 inches from the heat or grill for 4 to 5 minutes on each side, or until no longer pink in the center.

Spoon the yogurt sauce over the chicken. Garnish with the lime wedges.

2 tablespoons fresh lime juice

1 tablespoon olive oil

¼ teaspoon pepper

4 boneless, skinless chicken breast halves (about 4 ounces each), all visible fat discarded

4 ounces fat-free plain yogurt

1 tablespoon snipped fresh cilantro

1 tablespoon snipped fresh mint

½ teaspoon ground cumin

Cooking spray

1 medium lime, cut into 4 wedges (optional)

PER SERVING

calories 174	**cholesterol** 66 mg	**protein** 28 g	**dietary exchanges**
total fat 5.0 g	**sodium** 97 mg	**calcium** 77 mg	3 lean meat
saturated 1.0 g	**carbohydrates** 3 g	**potassium** 378 mg	
trans 0.0 g	fiber 0 g		
polyunsaturated 0.5 g	sugars 2 g		
monounsaturated 3.0 g			

BLACKBERRY-BALSAMIC CHICKEN

When the leaves start to change color, prepare this earthy dish of seared chicken breasts topped with a sauce made of blackberries, balsamic vinegar, and a hint of brown sugar and lemon zest.

SERVES 4 | 3 ounces chicken, ½ cup rice, and 2 tablespoons sauce per serving

Prepare the rice using the package directions for half the box, omitting the margarine. Remove from the heat. Cover to keep warm.

Meanwhile, sprinkle the seasoning blend over both sides of the chicken. Using your fingertips, gently press the seasoning blend so it adheres to the chicken.

In a large nonstick skillet, heat the oil over medium-high heat, swirling to coat the bottom. Cook the chicken for 4 minutes. Turn over and cook for 2 to 4 minutes, or until browned and no longer pink in the center. Transfer to a serving plate. Cover to keep warm.

In the same skillet, stir together the remaining ingredients. Cook over medium heat for 3 to 4 minutes, or until heated through, stirring occasionally. Stir in any accumulated juices from the chicken.

Serve the chicken with the rice on the side. Pour the sauce over all.

½ 6- to 7-ounce box quick-cooking white and wild rice, seasoning packet discarded

1 teaspoon salt-free all-purpose seasoning blend

4 boneless, skinless chicken breast halves (about 4 ounces each), flattened to ¼-inch thickness, or 1 pound turkey breast cutlets, all visible fat discarded (no need to flatten the turkey)

1 teaspoon olive oil

1 cup frozen unsweetened blackberries, thawed, juice reserved

¼ cup Chicken Broth (page 50) or commercial fat-free, low-sodium chicken broth

1 tablespoon light brown sugar

1 tablespoon balsamic vinegar

1 teaspoon grated lemon zest

COOK'S TIP If you prefer a seedless sauce, use a rubber scraper to press the sauce through a fine-mesh sieve into a medium bowl. This will yield about ¼ cup sauce (1 tablespoon per serving). If you want 2 tablespoons of strained sauce per serving, start with 2 cups frozen blackberries (thawed with juice). The remaining ingredient amounts stay the same.

COOK'S TIP ON FLATTENING CHICKEN BREASTS Flattening chicken breasts makes it easier to cook them uniformly. One way is to put a boneless, skinless chicken breast with the smooth side up between two pieces of plastic wrap. Using the smooth side of a meat mallet or a heavy pan, flatten the chicken to the desired thickness, being careful so you don't tear the meat.

PER SERVING

calories 266	**cholesterol** 66 mg	**protein** 29 g	**dietary exchanges**
total fat 2.5 g	**sodium** 80 mg	**calcium** 30 mg	1½ starch
saturated 0.5 g	**carbohydrates** 30 g	**potassium** 365 mg	½ fruit
trans 0.0 g	fiber 2 g		3 very lean meat
polyunsaturated 0.5 g	sugars 8 g		
monounsaturated 1.0 g			

HERB CHICKEN
with Panko-Pecan Crust

This fast-to-fix faux-fried entrée with its crunchy, herby crust is the perfect foundation to complement one of our sauces or salsas, such as Barbecue Sauce (page 265) or Roasted Tomato Chipotle Salsa (page 269). Pair this dish with Green Beans and Corn (page 236) or Greens with Tomatoes and Parmesan (page 245) to add color to the plate.

SERVES 4 | 3 ounces chicken per serving

Pour the buttermilk into a shallow dish.

In another shallow dish, stir together the panko, pecans, parsley, thyme, and pepper.

Set the dishes and a large plate in a row, assembly-line fashion. Dip the chicken in the buttermilk, turning to coat and letting the excess drip off. Dip in the panko mixture, turning to coat and gently shaking off any excess. Using your fingertips, gently press the mixture so it adheres to the chicken. Transfer the chicken to the plate. Lightly spray the top side of the chicken with cooking spray.

In a large nonstick skillet, heat the oil over medium-high heat, swirling to coat the bottom. Cook the chicken with the sprayed side down for 4 minutes. Turn over. Cook for 2 to 4 minutes, or until it is no longer pink in the center and the crust is golden brown.

½ cup low-fat buttermilk

¾ cup panko (Japanese bread crumbs)

3 tablespoons finely chopped pecans

1 teaspoon dried parsley, crumbled

½ teaspoon dried thyme, crumbled

¼ teaspoon pepper (coarsely ground preferred)

4 boneless, skinless chicken breast halves (about 4 ounces each), all visible fat discarded

Cooking spray

2 teaspoons olive oil

PER SERVING

calories 220	**cholesterol** 66 mg	**protein** 28 g	**dietary exchanges**
total fat 7.5 g	**sodium** 95 mg	**calcium** 37 mg	½ starch
saturated 1.0 g	**carbohydrates** 9 g	**potassium** 332 mg	3 lean meat
trans 0.0 g	fiber 1 g		
polyunsaturated 1.5 g	sugars 0 g		
monounsaturated 4.0 g			

CUMIN-LIME CHICKEN

This chicken dish makes its own sauce as it bakes, cutting down on the amount of work for you.

SERVES 4 | 3 ounces chicken and 3 tablespoons vegetable mixture per serving

Preheat the oven to 350°F. Lightly spray an 11 x 7 x 2-inch baking pan with cooking spray.

Place the chicken in a single layer in the pan. Squeeze the juice of ½ lime over the chicken. Sprinkle with the cumin. Top with the bell pepper and onion.

Bake for 28 to 30 minutes, or until the chicken is no longer pink in the center. Using a slotted spatula, transfer the chicken to plates.

Stir the tomato, cilantro, and salt into the pan, scraping to dislodge any browned bits. Squeeze the juice from the remaining ½ lime into the pan. Stir well. Spoon over the chicken. Top each serving with a dollop of sour cream.

Cooking spray

4 boneless, skinless chicken breast halves (about 4 ounces each), all visible fat discarded

1 medium lime, halved, divided use

1 teaspoon ground cumin

½ medium green bell pepper, finely chopped, or ½ cup finely chopped poblano pepper

¼ large onion, finely chopped

1 small tomato, chopped

2 tablespoons snipped fresh cilantro

¼ teaspoon salt

¼ cup fat-free sour cream

PER SERVING

calories 157	**cholesterol** 68 mg	**protein** 28 g	**dietary exchanges**
total fat 1.5 g	**sodium** 235 mg	**calcium** 56 mg	1 vegetable
saturated 0.5 g	**carbohydrates** 6 g	**potassium** 449 mg	3 very lean meat
trans 0.0 g	fiber 1 g		
polyunsaturated 0.5 g	sugars 3 g		
monounsaturated 0.5 g			

GRILLED SESAME CHICKEN

Sesame seeds give grilled chicken a crunchy difference your family will enjoy.

SERVES 4 | 3 ounces chicken per serving

Lightly spray the grill rack or broiler pan and rack with cooking spray. Preheat the grill on medium high or preheat the broiler.

Lightly season the chicken with the paprika and cayenne. Set aside on a large plate.

In a small microwaveable bowl, whisk together the lemon juice and honey. Microwave on 100 percent power (high) for 1 minute, or until the honey is dissolved.

Pour 2 tablespoons of the lemon juice mixture into a small bowl. Stir in the sesame seeds. Set aside to use as the sauce.

Coat the chicken with about 3 tablespoons of the remaining lemon juice mixture. Reserve the rest for basting.

Grill the chicken or broil 4 to 5 inches from the heat for 5 minutes, basting the top side occasionally with the reserved basting mixture (not the sauce). To prevent transferring harmful bacteria, wash the basting brush after each use. Turn the chicken over and cook for 5 to 6 minutes, or until no longer pink in the center, basting occasionally. Serve the chicken topped with the reserved sauce.

Cooking spray

4 boneless, skinless chicken breast halves (about 4 ounces each), all visible fat discarded

Paprika to taste

Cayenne to taste

¼ cup fresh lemon juice

¼ cup honey

1 tablespoon dry-roasted sesame seeds

PER SERVING

calories 207	**cholesterol** 66 mg	**protein** 27 g	**dietary exchanges**
total fat 3.0 g	**sodium** 76 mg	**calcium** 16 mg	1 other carbohydrate
saturated 0.5 g	**carbohydrates** 19 g	**potassium** 328 mg	3 very lean meat
trans 0.0 g	fiber 0 g		
polyunsaturated 1.0 g	sugars 18 g		
monounsaturated 1.0 g			

CREOLE CHICKEN STEW

Unlike many other stews, this one is quick enough for a weeknight. By the time instant brown rice finishes cooking, the stew is just about ready, too.

SERVES 4 | 1¼ cups stew and ½ cup rice per serving

In a small saucepan, stir together the rice and 1 cup water. Cook using the package directions, omitting the salt and margarine.

Meanwhile, in a medium bowl, stir together the paprika, pepper, and cayenne. Add the chicken cubes, stirring to coat.

In a large nonstick skillet, heat the oil over medium-high heat, swirling to coat the bottom. Cook the chicken for 5 minutes, stirring occasionally, until lightly browned (the chicken won't be done at this point). Transfer to a plate.

In the same skillet, cook the onion, bell pepper, and celery, still over medium-high heat, for 5 minutes, or until the vegetables begin to soften, stirring frequently.

Stir in the garlic. Cook for 1 minute, stirring constantly.

Stir in the tomatoes with liquid, oregano, salt, and chicken. Bring to a boil. Reduce the heat and simmer, covered, for 10 minutes, or until the chicken is no longer pink in the center and the sauce is slightly thickened. Serve the stew with the rice on the side.

- ½ cup uncooked instant brown rice
- 1 cup water
- 1 teaspoon paprika
- ¼ teaspoon pepper
- ⅛ teaspoon cayenne (optional)
- 1 pound boneless, skinless chicken breasts, all visible fat discarded, cut into 1-inch cubes
- 2 teaspoons olive oil
- 1 medium onion, chopped
- 1 medium green bell pepper, chopped
- 1 medium rib of celery, chopped
- 2 medium garlic cloves, minced
- 2 14.5-ounce cans no-salt-added diced tomatoes, undrained
- ½ teaspoon dried oregano, crumbled
- ¼ teaspoon salt

PER SERVING

calories 258	**cholesterol** 66 mg	**protein** 30 g	**dietary exchanges**
total fat 4.0 g	**sodium** 261 mg	**calcium** 69 mg	½ starch
saturated 0.5 g	**carbohydrates** 24 g	**potassium** 835 mg	3 vegetable
trans 0.0 g	fiber 4 g		3 lean meat
polyunsaturated 0.5 g	sugars 10 g		
monounsaturated 2.0 g			

ARROZ CON POLLO
(Chicken with Rice)

¡Delicioso! is what you'll be saying after you've enjoyed this Spanish-influenced one-dish meal.

SERVES 6 | scant 1¼ cups per serving

Preheat the oven to 350°F. Lightly spray a 13 x 9 x 2-inch casserole dish with cooking spray.

Put the chicken in the casserole dish.

In a small bowl, stir together the margarine, garlic, pepper, and paprika. Brush on the top side of the chicken.

Bake for 15 to 20 minutes, or until the chicken is no longer pink in the center.

Meanwhile, in a large nonstick skillet, heat the oil over medium-high heat, swirling to coat the bottom. Cook the onion and bell pepper for 3 to 4 minutes, or until soft, stirring frequently. Reduce the heat to medium.

Stir in the rice. Cook for 2 to 3 minutes, or until the rice begins to brown, stirring frequently.

Stir in the broth, tomatoes, and turmeric. Bring to a simmer. Simmer, covered, for 20 minutes.

Stir in the peas and chicken. Simmer, covered, for 10 minutes, or until heated through.

Cooking spray

1½ pounds boneless, skinless chicken breasts, all visible fat discarded, cut into bite-size pieces

1 tablespoon light tub margarine, melted

1 medium garlic clove, minced

¼ teaspoon pepper

¼ teaspoon paprika

1 teaspoon olive oil

½ to 1 small onion, chopped

¼ medium green bell pepper, chopped

1 cup uncooked rice

2 cups Chicken Broth (page 50) or commercial fat-free, low-sodium chicken broth

2 medium tomatoes, chopped

⅛ teaspoon turmeric

1 cup frozen green peas

PER SERVING

calories 275	**cholesterol** 66 mg	**protein** 31 g	**dietary exchanges**
total fat 3.0 g	**sodium** 124 mg	**calcium** 29 mg	2 starch
saturated 0.5 g	**carbohydrates** 30 g	**potassium** 493 mg	3 very lean meat
trans 0.0 g	fiber 2 g		
polyunsaturated 0.5 g	sugars 3 g		
monounsaturated 1.5 g			

CHICKEN PAPRIKASH

Richly colored with paprika, this traditional Hungarian entrée is full bodied and satisfying. It goes well with Balsamic-Marinated Vegetables (page 78).

SERVES 6 | 1 cup per serving

Prepare the pasta using the package directions, omitting the salt. Drain well in a colander.

Meanwhile, lightly spray a large skillet with cooking spray. Heat over medium-high heat. Cook the chicken for 4 minutes, or until lightly browned on all sides, stirring occasionally. Transfer to a plate. Reduce the heat to medium.

In the same skillet, stir together the onion and paprika. Cook for 3 minutes, or until the onion is soft, stirring constantly. Stir in the tomato and broth. Cook for 2 minutes, or until hot.

Return the chicken to the skillet. Bring to a simmer. Reduce the heat and simmer, covered, for 30 minutes, or until the chicken is no longer pink in the center. Using a slotted spoon, transfer the chicken, onion, and tomato to another plate. Set aside.

Sprinkle the flour over the broth mixture remaining in the skillet. Cook for 2 to 3 minutes, or until the sauce has thickened, whisking constantly.

In a small bowl, whisk together the yogurt and sour cream. Whisk into the sauce. Stir in the chicken mixture. Serve over the pasta.

2½ cups dried no-yolk noodles

Cooking spray

1½ pounds boneless, skinless chicken breasts, all visible fat discarded, cut into bite-size pieces

1 medium red onion, thinly sliced

2 tablespoons paprika (sweet Hungarian paprika preferred)

1 medium tomato, chopped

½ cup Chicken Broth (page 50) or commercial fat-free, low-sodium chicken broth

2 tablespoons all-purpose flour

½ cup fat-free plain yogurt

2 tablespoons fat-free sour cream

PER SERVING

calories 238	**cholesterol** 67 mg	**protein** 31 g	**dietary exchanges**
total fat 2.0 g	**sodium** 108 mg	**calcium** 80 mg	1½ starch
saturated 0.5 g	**carbohydrates** 22 g	**potassium** 524 mg	3 very lean meat
trans 0.0 g	fiber 2 g		
polyunsaturated 0.5 g	sugars 5 g		
monounsaturated 0.5 g			

SLOW-COOKER MOROCCAN CHICKEN with Orange Couscous

Thanks to a wonderful blend of spices and dried fruit, ordinary chicken gets a Moroccan makeover in this meal-in-one dish. Don't be put off by the long list of ingredients—this dish is simple to put together.

SERVES 6 | 1 cup chicken mixture and ½ cup couscous per serving

Lightly spray a 3½- or 4-quart slow cooker with cooking spray. Put the carrots, onion, and celery in the slow cooker. Place the chicken cubes over the vegetables. Top with the dried plums, apricots, and raisins. Don't stir.

In a medium bowl, whisk together the vinegar and flour until smooth. Gradually whisk in the wine. Whisk in the remaining chicken ingredients except the beans. Pour over the chicken mixture. Don't stir. Cook, covered, on low for 5½ to 6½ hours or on high for 2½ to 3 hours, or until the chicken and vegetables are tender. Stir in the beans. Cook, covered, for 5 to 10 minutes (on either low or high), or until the beans are heated through.

Cooking spray

CHICKEN

- 2 medium carrots, cut crosswise into ½-inch pieces
- 1 medium sweet onion, such as Vidalia, Maui, or Oso Sweet, halved lengthwise, thinly sliced lengthwise, and separated into half-rings
- 1 large rib of celery, chopped
- 1 pound boneless, skinless chicken breasts, all visible fat discarded, cut into 1½- to 2-inch cubes
- ⅓ cup dried plums, coarsely chopped
- ⅓ cup dried apricots, coarsely chopped
- ⅓ cup golden raisins
- ⅓ cup white balsamic vinegar
- 2 tablespoons all-purpose flour
- 1 cup dry white wine (regular or nonalcoholic)

(continued)

While the beans are heating, in a small saucepan, bring the water and orange juice just to a boil over high heat. Remove from the heat. Stir in the couscous. Let stand, covered, for 5 minutes. Fluff with a fork. Spoon onto plates. Ladle the chicken mixture over the couscous mixture.

3 tablespoons firmly packed light brown sugar

3 medium garlic cloves, minced

1 teaspoon ground cumin

1 teaspoon ground ginger

1 teaspoon ground cinnamon

¼ teaspoon cayenne

1 15.5-ounce can no-salt-added cannellini beans, white kidney beans, or chickpeas, rinsed and drained

COUSCOUS

½ cup water

½ cup fresh orange juice

1 cup uncooked whole-wheat couscous

PER SERVING

calories 450	**cholesterol** 44 mg	**protein** 28 g	**dietary exchanges**
total fat 2.5 g	**sodium** 108 mg	**calcium** 99 mg	3 starch
saturated 0.5 g	**carbohydrates** 76 g	**potassium** 833 mg	1½ fruit
trans 0.0 g	fiber 11 g		1 vegetable
polyunsaturated 0.5 g	sugars 27 g		2½ very lean meat
monounsaturated 0.5 g			

LEMON CHICKEN
with Oregano

Lots of fresh seasonings make this stovetop entrée sparkle. Try it with steamed brown rice and Greens with Tomatoes and Parmesan (page 245) on the side.

SERVES 4 | 3 ounces chicken per serving

Lightly spray a large skillet with cooking spray. Add the oil, lemon zest, and lemon juice, swirling to coat the bottom. Stir in the chicken, oregano, garlic, and pepper. Cook, covered, over medium-high heat for 3 to 5 minutes, or until the chicken begins to turn white. Turn the chicken over. Cook for 3 to 5 minutes, or until the entire surface is white. Pour the pan liquid into a small bowl to reserve.

Cook the chicken, uncovered, for 2 to 5 minutes on each side, or until lightly browned.

Sprinkle the paprika over the chicken. Pour the reserved pan liquid into the skillet. Cook for 3 to 5 minutes, or until the chicken is no longer pink in the center, stirring frequently. Serve sprinkled with the parsley.

Cooking spray

- 2 teaspoons canola or corn oil
- ½ teaspoon grated lemon zest
- 2 tablespoons fresh lemon juice
- 1 pound chicken breast tenders, all visible fat discarded
- 2 to 3 tablespoons chopped fresh oregano or 2 to 3 teaspoons dried, crumbled
- 1 medium garlic clove, minced
- ⅛ teaspoon pepper
- ¼ teaspoon paprika
- 2 tablespoons snipped fresh parsley

PER SERVING

calories 152	**cholesterol** 66 mg	**protein** 26 g	**dietary exchanges**
total fat 4.0 g	**sodium** 75 mg	**calcium** 29 mg	3 lean meat
saturated 0.5 g	**carbohydrates** 2 g	**potassium** 329 mg	
trans 0.0 g	fiber 0 g		
polyunsaturated 1.0 g	sugars 0 g		
monounsaturated 2.0 g			

CHICKEN
with Ginger and Snow Peas

Serve this Asian-inspired dish with a colorful fruit salad and soba noodles.

SERVES 5 | 1 cup per serving

Put the cornstarch in a small bowl. Add ½ cup broth, the soy sauce, and pepper, whisking to dissolve the cornstarch. Set aside.

In a large, heavy skillet, heat the oil over high heat, swirling to coat the bottom. Cook the chicken for 4 minutes, stirring frequently.

Stir in the snow peas, garlic, and gingerroot. Cook for 3 minutes, stirring constantly.

Add the broth mixture. Cook for 2 to 3 minutes, or until the sauce thickens and the chicken is no longer pink in the center, stirring constantly. If the mixture begins to burn, remove from the heat for a moment or stir in the remaining 1 to 2 tablespoons broth.

1 tablespoon cornstarch

½ cup Chicken Broth (page 50) or commercial fat-free, low-sodium chicken broth, and 1 to 2 tablespoons Chicken Broth (page 50) or commercial fat-free, low-sodium chicken broth, if needed, divided use

1 tablespoon soy sauce (lowest sodium available)

1 teaspoon pepper

2 teaspoons canola or corn oil

1¼ pounds chicken breast tenders, all visible fat discarded

6 ounces snow peas, trimmed

2 medium garlic cloves, minced

½ teaspoon minced peeled gingerroot

PER SERVING

calories 168	**cholesterol** 66 mg	**protein** 28 g	**dietary exchanges**
total fat 3.5 g	**sodium** 157 mg	**calcium** 32 mg	1 vegetable
saturated 0.5 g	**carbohydrates** 5 g	**potassium** 388 mg	3 very lean meat
trans 0.0 g	fiber 1 g		
polyunsaturated 1.0 g	sugars 1 g		
monounsaturated 1.5 g			

CHICKEN PRIMAVERA

Simmer spring vegetables and chunks of chicken in a rich tomato sauce to serve over whole-grain fettuccine. Round out the meal with a seasonal fresh fruit salad.

SERVES 8 | 1 cup pasta and ¾ cup chicken mixture per serving

In a large saucepan, heat the oil over medium heat, swirling to coat the bottom. Cook the zucchini, yellow squash, onion, mushrooms, and garlic for 3 to 4 minutes, or until the squashes and onion are tender-crisp, stirring occasionally.

Stir in the tomatoes with liquid, broth, oregano, pepper, and red pepper flakes. Increase the heat to medium high and bring to a simmer. Reduce the heat to medium low and cook for 15 minutes, stirring occasionally.

Meanwhile, prepare the pasta using the package directions, omitting the salt. Drain well in a colander. Pour into a large bowl and cover to keep warm.

Stir the chicken and peas into the zucchini mixture. Increase the heat to medium and cook for 5 to 10 minutes, or until the chicken and peas are heated through, stirring occasionally. Serve over the pasta.

1 teaspoon olive oil

1 medium zucchini, chopped

1 medium yellow summer squash, chopped

1 medium red onion, chopped

2 ounces mushrooms, such as cremini (brown), sliced

2 medium garlic cloves, minced

1 14.5-ounce can no-salt-added diced tomatoes, undrained

½ cup Chicken Broth (page 50) or commercial fat-free, low-sodium chicken broth

1 teaspoon dried oregano, crumbled

¼ teaspoon pepper

¼ teaspoon crushed red pepper flakes

16 ounces dried whole-grain fettuccine

(continued)

COOK'S TIP Use this recipe as a springboard for experimentation. A few possibilities are using asparagus for one or both types of squash, substituting green onions for red, trying thyme instead of oregano, and/or replacing the fettuccine with whole-grain bowtie pasta.

COOK'S TIP ON CANNED TOMATOES Cooking with no-salt-added tomatoes can really make a difference in sodium: On average, one cup of regular canned tomatoes contains 300 mg more than the same amount of tomatoes canned without added salt!

2 cups cubed cooked skinless chicken breasts, cooked without salt, all visible fat discarded

1 cup frozen green peas

PER SERVING

calories 299
total fat 3.0 g
  saturated 0.5 g
  trans 0.0 g
  polyunsaturated 1.0 g
  monounsaturated 1.0 g

cholesterol 30 mg
sodium 59 mg
carbohydrates 51 g
  fiber 10 g
  sugars 6 g

protein 22 g
calcium 64 mg
potassium 522 mg

dietary exchanges
3 starch
1 vegetable
1½ very lean meat

CHICKEN, BARLEY, AND SPINACH CASSEROLE

Full of healthy ingredients, this wonderfully comforting almond-topped casserole will wow even spinach-phobes.

SERVES 4 | 1½ cups per serving

Preheat the oven to 350°F. Lightly spray a 2-quart glass casserole dish with cooking spray. Set aside.

In a large saucepan, heat the oil over medium-high heat, swirling to coat the bottom. Cook the onion, carrot, and garlic for 3 minutes, or until the onion is soft, stirring frequently.

Stir in the mushrooms. Cook for 3 minutes, or until soft, stirring frequently.

Stir in the chicken, water, bouillon, and pepper. Cook, covered, for 2 minutes, or until the mixture reaches a boil.

Stir in the barley. Reduce the heat and simmer, covered, for 10 to 12 minutes, or until the barley is tender and the water has almost been absorbed. Remove from the heat.

Stir in the spinach. Spoon into the casserole dish. Sprinkle with the almonds.

Bake for 15 minutes, or until heated through.

Cooking spray
- 2 teaspoons olive oil
- 1 medium onion, chopped
- 1 medium carrot, finely chopped
- 2 medium garlic cloves, minced
- 1½ cups sliced mushrooms, any variety or combination
- 1 pound boneless, skinless chicken breasts, cooked without salt, all visible fat discarded, cut into ½-inch cubes
- 2 cups water
- 1 teaspoon sodium-free powdered chicken bouillon
- ½ teaspoon pepper
- 1 cup uncooked quick-cooking barley
- 10 ounces frozen chopped spinach, thawed, drained, and squeezed until very dry
- 2 tablespoons sliced almonds, dry-roasted

PER SERVING

calories 338	**cholesterol** 66 mg	**protein** 35 g	**dietary exchanges**
total fat 6.5 g	**sodium** 148 mg	**calcium** 146 mg	2 starch
saturated 1.0 g	**carbohydrates** 38 g	**potassium** 1019 mg	2 vegetable
trans 0.0 g	fiber 8 g		3 lean meat
polyunsaturated 1.5 g	sugars 4 g		
monounsaturated 3.0 g			

TARRAGON TURKEY MEDALLIONS

Preparation of this entrée is very fast paced, so have your side dishes ready before you begin cooking it. Mixed salad greens topped with Cider Vinaigrette (page 96) and Rice and Vegetable Pilaf (page 252) make good accompaniments.

SERVES 4 | 3 ounces turkey per serving

In a small bowl, whisk together the sauce ingredients. Set aside.

Lightly spray a large skillet with cooking spray. Heat the oil over high heat, swirling to coat the bottom. Cook the turkey in a single layer for 2 minutes. Turn over and cook for 3 minutes, or until no longer pink in the center. Transfer to a serving plate. Set aside.

Pour the sauce into the skillet. Cook for 15 to 20 seconds, or until the mixture reduces to 2 tablespoons, stirring constantly with a flat spatula. Drizzle over the turkey.

SAUCE
- 2 tablespoons fresh lemon juice
- 2 tablespoons water
- 1½ teaspoons fresh tarragon or ½ teaspoon dried, crumbled
- 1 medium garlic clove, minced
- ¼ teaspoon salt
- ⅛ teaspoon pepper

Cooking spray
- 2 teaspoons olive oil
- 1 1-pound turkey tenderloin, all visible fat discarded, cut crosswise into ¼-inch slices

COOK'S TIP Substitute a 1-pound pork tenderloin for the turkey. Cook as directed above.

PER SERVING

calories 149	**cholesterol** 70 mg	**protein** 28 g	**dietary exchanges**
total fat 3.0 g	**sodium** 202 mg	**calcium** 15 mg	3 very lean meat
saturated 0.5 g	**carbohydrates** 1 g	**potassium** 349 mg	
trans 0.0 g	fiber 0 g		
polyunsaturated 0.5 g	sugars 0 g		
monounsaturated 2.0 g			

TURKEY TENDERLOIN
with Rosemary

With this recipe, you season and bake a turkey tenderloin, then make a sauce—all in one dish. It's a great entrée to serve when you're in a hurry and even greater when you're the one cleaning up.

SERVES 4 | 3 ounces turkey per serving

Preheat the oven to 350°F. Lightly spray a large glass baking dish with cooking spray.

Put the oil, rosemary, lemon juice, lemon pepper, and garlic in the baking dish, stirring to combine. Add the turkey, turning to coat. Tuck the ends under for even cooking.

Bake for 20 minutes. Turn over and bake for 20 to 25 minutes, or until the turkey registers 160°F on an instant-read thermometer. Transfer the turkey to a cutting board, retaining the liquid in the baking dish and leaving the oven on. Let the turkey stand for 5 minutes to continue cooking (it should reach at least 165°F). Thinly slice diagonally across the grain. Arrange the sliced turkey on a serving plate.

Meanwhile, pour the broth and wine into the baking dish, scraping to dislodge any browned bits. Stir well. Return the baking dish to the oven for 3 to 4 minutes, or until the broth is heated through. Pour the sauce over the turkey slices.

Cooking spray
- 1 tablespoon olive oil
- 1 tablespoon chopped fresh rosemary or 1 teaspoon dried, crushed
- 1 teaspoon fresh lemon juice
- ¾ teaspoon salt-free lemon pepper
- 1 medium garlic clove, minced
- 1 1-pound turkey tenderloin, all visible fat discarded
- ¼ cup Chicken Broth (page 50) or commercial fat-free, low-sodium chicken broth
- 1 tablespoon dry white wine (regular or nonalcoholic)

PORK TENDERLOIN
with Rosemary

Substitute a 1-pound pork tenderloin for the turkey. Roast for 20 to 25 minutes, or until the pork registers 150°F on an instant-read thermometer, or is slightly pink in the very center. Transfer the pork to a cutting board. Let stand for about 10 minutes before slicing. The pork will continue to cook during the standing time, reaching about 160°F.

COOK'S TIP ON FRESH ROSEMARY Sprigs of rosemary are hardy and will keep for about two weeks in an airtight plastic bag in the refrigerator.

PER SERVING

calories 162	**cholesterol** 70 mg	**protein** 28 g	**dietary exchanges**
total fat 4.0 g	**sodium** 58 mg	**calcium** 19 mg	3 lean meat
saturated 0.5 g	**carbohydrates** 1 g	**potassium** 355 mg	
trans 0.0 g	fiber 0 g		
polyunsaturated 0.5 g	sugars 0 g		
monounsaturated 2.5 g			

PER SERVING
PORK TENDERLOIN WITH ROSEMARY

calories 159	**cholesterol** 74 mg	**protein** 24 g	**dietary exchanges**
total fat 6.0 g	**sodium** 62 mg	**calcium** 13 mg	3 lean meat
saturated 1.5 g	**carbohydrates** 1 g	**potassium** 475 mg	
trans 0.0 g	fiber 0 g		
polyunsaturated 1.0 g	sugars 0 g		
monounsaturated 3.5 g			

ROASTED LEMON-HERB TURKEY BREAST

Fresh lemon, fresh parsley, and lots of dried herbs tucked between the skin and the meat infuse this turkey with sensational flavors. If there is leftover turkey, you can use it in Turkey Stew (page 167).

SERVES 12 | 3 ounces turkey per serving

Preheat the oven to 325°F. Lightly spray a roasting pan and baking rack with cooking spray.

Cut the lemons in half. Squeeze about ¼ cup juice into a small bowl. Set aside the lemon halves.

Whisk the parsley, basil, mustard, oil, oregano, pepper, and garlic powder into the lemon juice.

Using a tablespoon or your fingers, carefully separate the skin from the meat of the turkey. Spread the lemon juice mixture between the skin and meat over as much area as possible, being careful not to tear the skin. Gently pull the skin over the top and sides. Put the turkey on the rack in the pan. Put the lemon halves in the pan, directly under the turkey. Sprinkle the top of the turkey with the paprika.

Cooking spray

2 medium lemons

½ cup snipped fresh parsley

1 tablespoon dried basil, crumbled

1 tablespoon Dijon mustard (lowest sodium available)

1 tablespoon olive oil

2 teaspoons dried oregano, crumbled

½ teaspoon pepper (coarsely ground preferred)

¼ teaspoon garlic powder

1 5-pound turkey breast with skin

Paprika to taste

Roast the turkey for 1 hour 30 minutes to 1 hour 45 minutes, or until the thickest part of the breast registers about 155°F on an instant-read thermometer. Remove from the oven and lightly cover. Let stand for 15 minutes to continue cooking (the breast should reach at least 165°F) and for easier slicing. Discard the skin and lemons before slicing the turkey.

PER SERVING

calories 181

total fat 2.0 g
  saturated 0.5 g
  trans 0.0 g
  polyunsaturated 0.5 g
  monounsaturated 1.0 g

cholesterol 93 mg
sodium 100 mg
carbohydrates 1 g
  fiber 0 g
  sugars 0 g

protein 37 g
calcium 29 mg
potassium 475 mg

dietary exchanges
4 very lean meat

TURKEY SAUSAGE PATTIES

These flavorful patties are a leaner version of the breakfast staple. Serve them with Pancakes (page 290) or Blueberry Muffins (page 285).

SERVES 4 | 1 patty per serving

Preheat the broiler. Lightly spray a broiler pan and rack with cooking spray.

In a medium bowl, using your hands or a spoon, combine the ingredients for the patties. Shape into 4 patties. Put the patties on the rack in the pan.

Broil the patties 2 to 4 inches from the heat for 10 minutes. Turn over and broil for 5 to 10 minutes, or until no longer pink in the center.

COOK'S TIP ON ALLSPICE The berry of the evergreen pimiento tree and native to the West Indies and South America, allspice is so named because it tastes like a combination of cinnamon, nutmeg, and cloves. Use allspice for a piquant flavor in foods from soups, stews, and meats to cakes and fruit dishes.

Cooking spray

PATTIES

- 12 ounces ground skinless turkey breast
- 1 large egg white
- 2 tablespoons water
- ¼ teaspoon pepper
- ¼ teaspoon dried basil, crumbled
- ¼ teaspoon dried sage
- ¼ teaspoon dried oregano, crumbled
- ⅛ teaspoon ground allspice
- ⅛ teaspoon ground nutmeg
- ⅛ teaspoon dried dillweed, crumbled
- ⅛ teaspoon garlic powder
- ⅛ teaspoon Chili Powder (page 277) or no-salt-added chili powder (optional)
- ⅛ teaspoon red hot-pepper sauce (optional)

PER SERVING

calories 101	**cholesterol** 53 mg	**protein** 22 g	**dietary exchanges**
total fat 0.5 g	**sodium** 56 mg	**calcium** 15 mg	3 very lean meat
saturated 0.0 g	**carbohydrates** 1 g	**potassium** 274 mg	
trans 0.0 g	fiber 0 g		
polyunsaturated 0.0 g	sugars 0 g		
monounsaturated 0.0 g			

TURKEY STEW

If you're wondering what to do with leftover holiday turkey, use it in this one-pot dish for the perfect post-holiday meal.

SERVES 8 | 1½ cups per serving

In a stockpot, heat the oil over medium-high heat, swirling to coat the bottom. Cook the onion for 3 minutes, or until soft, stirring frequently.

Pour in the broth. Bring to a boil, stirring occasionally.

In a small bowl, whisk together the water and flour. Whisk into the broth mixture. Cook for 5 minutes, or until the broth just begins to thicken, whisking constantly.

Stir in the turkey, celery, carrots, poultry seasoning, bay leaf, garlic powder, and pepper. Bring to a boil. Reduce the heat and simmer for 15 minutes, or until heated through.

Stir in the potatoes. Cook, covered, for 30 minutes, or until the celery, carrots, and potatoes are tender, stirring occasionally.

Stir in the peas. Cook for 5 minutes. Discard the bay leaf before serving the stew.

2 teaspoons canola or corn oil

1 medium onion, chopped

4 cups Chicken Broth (page 50) or commercial fat-free, low-sodium chicken broth

¼ cup water

2 tablespoons all-purpose flour

1¼ pounds cooked turkey breast, cooked without salt, skin and all visible fat discarded, cut into bite-size pieces

6 medium ribs of celery, coarsely chopped

6 medium carrots, coarsely chopped

1 teaspoon poultry seasoning

1 medium dried bay leaf

½ teaspoon garlic powder

¼ to ½ teaspoon pepper

6 medium potatoes, coarsely chopped

1½ cups frozen green peas

PER SERVING

calories 301	**cholesterol** 61 mg	**protein** 28 g	**dietary exchanges**
total fat 2.5 g	**sodium** 150 mg	**calcium** 77 mg	2½ starch
saturated 0.5 g	**carbohydrates** 42 g	**potassium** 1232 mg	1 vegetable
trans 0.0 g	fiber 6 g		3 very lean meat
polyunsaturated 0.5 g	sugars 7 g		
monounsaturated 1.0 g			

TURKEY AND BROCCOLI STIR-FRY

When you've had enough sandwiches made of leftover turkey, try this colorful stir-fry.

SERVES 4 | 1½ cups per serving

In a medium saucepan, prepare the rice using the package directions, omitting the salt and margarine.

Meanwhile, lightly spray a large skillet with cooking spray. Cook the bell pepper and onion over medium-high heat for 5 minutes, or until they begin to lightly brown on the edges, stirring frequently. Transfer to a plate. Set aside.

Pour the water into the skillet. Stir in the broccoli. Cook for 2 minutes, or until the broccoli is just tender-crisp, stirring constantly.

Stir in the bell pepper mixture and turkey. Remove from the heat. Let stand, covered, for 3 minutes, or until the turkey is heated through.

Meanwhile, in a small microwaveable bowl, whisk together the remaining ingredients. Microwave on 100 percent power (high) for 20 seconds, or until hot.

Spoon the rice onto plates. Spoon the turkey mixture over the rice. Top with the sauce.

1 cup uncooked quick-cooking brown rice

Cooking spray

½ medium red bell pepper, cut into thin strips

½ large onion, thinly sliced

¼ cup water

2 cups small broccoli florets

2 cups diced cooked turkey breast, cooked without salt, skin and all visible fat discarded

3 tablespoons hoisin sauce

2 tablespoons honey

2 to 3 teaspoons fresh lime juice

1 teaspoon toasted sesame oil

PER SERVING

calories 271	**cholesterol** 60 mg	**protein** 25 g	**dietary exchanges**
total fat 3.0 g	**sodium** 122 mg	**calcium** 41 mg	1 starch
saturated 0.5 g	**carbohydrates** 36 g	**potassium** 439 mg	1 other carbohydrate
trans 0.0 g	fiber 3 g		1 vegetable
polyunsaturated 1.0 g	sugars 15 g		3 very lean meat
monounsaturated 1.0 g			

MEATS

EASY ROAST BEEF

You'll be transported back to Grandma's kitchen when you smell this homey dish as it cooks. The leftovers are excellent for sandwiches and recipes calling for cooked lean beef, such as Vegetable Beef Soup (page 68).

SERVES 18 | 3 ounces beef per serving

Preheat the oven to 350°F. Lightly spray a roasting pan with olive oil spray. Set aside.

Rub the beef on all sides with the oil. Sprinkle with the Chili Powder. Using your fingertips, gently press the Chili Powder so it adheres to the beef. Transfer the beef to the roasting pan. Put the onion, carrots, and celery around the beef.

In a small bowl, stir together the wine and Worcestershire sauce. Pour over the beef.

Bake for 1 hour 30 minutes, or until a meat thermometer inserted in the thickest part of the beef registers almost the desired doneness. If the beef begins to dry out during cooking, baste with additional wine. Don't use the drippings for basting. Leaving the pan juices in the pan, transfer the beef to a cutting board, retaining the pan juices. Let stand, lightly covered with aluminum foil, for 10 to 15 minutes to continue cooking. Thinly slice the beef. Arrange on a platter.

Olive oil spray
- 1 5-pound beef rump roast, all visible fat discarded
- 2 tablespoons olive oil
- 1 tablespoon Chili Powder (page 277) or no-salt-added chili powder
- 1 medium onion, thinly sliced
- 2 medium carrots, thinly sliced
- 1 large rib of celery, thinly sliced
- ½ cup dry red wine (regular or nonalcoholic) (plus more as needed)
- 1 tablespoon Worcestershire sauce (lowest sodium available)
- ½ teaspoon salt

Meanwhile, skim the fat from the pan juices or remove the juices with a bulb baster and discard the fat. Stir the salt into the pan juices. Spoon over the sliced beef.

COOK'S TIP ON BEEF TEMPERATURES Use a meat thermometer or an instant-read thermometer to determine the internal temperature. To be safe, cook beef to at least 160°F. For well-done, cook to 170°F.

COOK'S TIP ON SEPARATING FAT FROM PAN JUICES A gravy separator, which looks like a measuring cup with a spout coming from the bottom, makes it easy to remove the fat from pan juices. Pour all the pan juices into the separator. After the fat rises to the top, simply pour the fat-free juice out of the bottom until the fat layer falls to the level of the spout. Discard what remains in the separator.

PER SERVING

calories 178	**cholesterol** 63 mg	**protein** 28 g	**dietary exchanges**
total fat 5.0 g	**sodium** 110 mg	**calcium** 12 mg	3 lean meat
saturated 1.5 g	**carbohydrates** 2 g	**potassium** 255 mg	
trans 0.0 g	fiber 1 g		
polyunsaturated 0.5 g	sugars 1 g		
monounsaturated 3.0 g			

BEEF BOURGUIGNON

Even though this fancy-sounding stew (pronounced *boor-gen-YUN* or *boor-ge-NYON*) takes a while to prepare, it's well worth the time. Packed with beef and vegetables, it's a complete meal in a bowl.

SERVES 8 | 1 cup per serving

In a large bowl, stir together the flour and pepper. Add the beef, turning to coat and shaking off the excess.

Lightly spray a Dutch oven with cooking spray. Heat the oil over medium-high heat, swirling to coat the bottom. Cook the beef for 1 to 2 minutes, stirring frequently.

Stir in the onion and garlic. Cook for 3 minutes, or until soft, stirring frequently.

Stir in the mushrooms. Cook for 1 to 2 minutes, or until they absorb the liquid in the pot.

Stir in the tomatoes, water, wine, and herb seasoning blend. Reduce the heat and simmer, covered, for 2 hours, stirring occasionally and adding water if needed to keep the bottom of the pot covered.

Stir in the potatoes and carrots. Simmer, covered, for 30 minutes, or until the beef and vegetables are tender.

2 tablespoons all-purpose flour

Pepper to taste

1 pound boneless lean beef chuck roast, all visible fat discarded, cut into 1-inch cubes

Cooking spray

1 teaspoon canola or corn oil

¼ cup chopped onion

1 medium garlic clove, minced

1 pound small whole button mushrooms

3 medium tomatoes, finely chopped, or 1 14.5-ounce can no-salt-added diced tomatoes, undrained

1½ cups water (plus more as needed)

½ cup dry red wine (regular or nonalcoholic)

1½ tablespoons salt-free herb seasoning blend

4 medium potatoes, peeled and coarsely diced (about 3 cups)

4 medium carrots, coarsely diced

SLOW-COOKER METHOD

Omit the cooking spray and oil. Put the coated beef cubes in a 3½- or 4-quart slow cooker. Add the remaining ingredients and cook, covered, on high for 4 to 5 hours or on low for 8 to 9 hours, or until the beef and vegetables are tender.

COOK'S TIP If you prefer, replace the herb seasoning blend with a combination of 1 tablespoon snipped fresh parsley; ¼ teaspoon dried thyme, crumbled; ¼ teaspoon dried basil, crumbled; ¼ teaspoon dried oregano, crumbled; ⅛ teaspoon dried rosemary, crushed; and ⅛ teaspoon dried marjoram, crumbled.

PER SERVING

calories 174	**cholesterol** 22 mg	**protein** 15 g	**dietary exchanges**
total fat 3.0 g	**sodium** 50 mg	**calcium** 42 mg	1 starch
saturated 1.0 g	**carbohydrates** 23 g	**potassium** 822 mg	2 vegetable
trans 0.0 g	fiber 3 g		1½ lean meat
polyunsaturated 0.5 g	sugars 5 g		
monounsaturated 1.5 g			

FRENCH COUNTRY SIRLOIN

Add a touch of Provence by applying a rub of thyme, marjoram, rosemary, and sage to sirloin steak.

SERVES 4 | 3 ounces beef per serving

Preheat the grill on medium high.

Using your fingertips, rub the oil on both sides of the beef.

In a small bowl, stir together the thyme, marjoram, rosemary, sage, pepper, and salt. Sprinkle over the beef. Gently press the mixture so it adheres to the beef.

Grill the beef, covered, for 6 to 8 minutes on each side, or until the desired doneness. After the first 5 minutes, put the tomatoes and green onions on the grill. Grill, covered, for 8 to 10 minutes, or until slightly charred, turning several times to cook evenly.

When the beef is done, transfer to a large plate. Cover the plate and set aside. When the tomatoes and green onions are done, transfer to a cutting board and coarsely chop. Spoon over the beef.

1 teaspoon olive oil

1 1-pound boneless sirloin steak, about 1 inch thick, all visible fat discarded, cut into 4 pieces

1 teaspoon dried thyme, crumbled

½ teaspoon dried marjoram, crumbled

½ teaspoon crushed dried rosemary

½ teaspoon dried sage

½ teaspoon pepper

¼ teaspoon salt

2 medium Italian plum (Roma) tomatoes, halved lengthwise

4 medium green onions

PER SERVING

calories 169	cholesterol 56 mg	protein 24 g	dietary exchanges
total fat 5.5 g	sodium 200 mg	calcium 17 mg	3 lean meat
saturated 2.0 g	carbohydrates 4 g	potassium 440 mg	
trans 0.0 g	fiber 2 g		
polyunsaturated 0.5 g	sugars 2 g		
monounsaturated 3.0 g			

SIRLOIN with Red Wine and Mushroom Sauce

A delicately sweet reduction of red wine, mushrooms, tomato sauce, and herbs crowns tender beef slices.

SERVES 4 | 3 ounces beef and ¼ cup sauce per serving

In a large shallow glass dish, stir together the mushrooms and wine. Add the beef, turning to coat. Cover and refrigerate for 8 to 12 hours, turning occasionally.

In a small bowl, stir together the tomato sauce, green onions, bouillon granules, basil, sugar, oregano, garlic powder, and salt. Set aside.

Lightly spray a large skillet with cooking spray. Heat over medium-high heat. Drain the beef well, reserving the marinade. Cook the beef for 4 minutes. Turn over. Cook for 2 minutes, or to the desired doneness. Transfer to a cutting board. Set aside.

Pour the reserved marinade and the tomato sauce mixture into the skillet, scraping the bottom and side to dislodge any browned bits. Cook over medium-high heat for 3 minutes, or until the liquid is reduced to 1 cup, stirring occasionally. Remove from the heat.

Slice the beef and transfer to plates. Spoon the mushroom sauce over the beef. Sprinkle with the parsley.

5 ounces medium button mushrooms, sliced

⅓ cup merlot or other dry red wine (regular or nonalcoholic)

1 1-pound boneless top sirloin steak (about 1 inch thick), all visible fat discarded

½ cup no-salt-added tomato sauce

2 medium green onions, finely chopped

1 teaspoon very low sodium beef bouillon granules

1 teaspoon dried basil, crumbled

¾ teaspoon sugar

½ teaspoon dried oregano, crumbled

⅛ teaspoon garlic powder

⅛ teaspoon salt

Cooking spray

2 tablespoons snipped fresh parsley

PER SERVING

calories 190	**cholesterol** 56 mg	**protein** 25 g	**dietary exchanges**
total fat 4.5 g	**sodium** 131 mg	**calcium** 24 mg	1 vegetable
saturated 2.0 g	**carbohydrates** 7 g	**potassium** 731 mg	3 lean meat
trans 0.0 g	fiber 2 g		
polyunsaturated 0.5 g	sugars 4 g		
monounsaturated 2.0 g			

BROILED SIRLOIN
with Chile-Roasted Onions

Sweet and mildly spicy roasted onions take steak to a new flavor level. Make a double batch of the onions (you can cover and refrigerate the extras for up to four days) and serve half with pork chops, such as Pork Chops with Herb Rub (page 196) or on open-face roast beef sandwiches. The steak needs to marinate for 8 hours, so be sure to plan accordingly.

SERVES 4 | 3 ounces beef and ¼ cup onions per serving

In a shallow glass dish, stir together the wine, 1 tablespoon brown sugar, and 1 teaspoon chili garlic sauce or paste until the sugar is dissolved. Add the beef, turning to coat. Cover and refrigerate for 8 hours, turning occasionally.

Preheat the oven to 400°F. Lightly spray a large shallow metal baking pan with cooking spray.

Spread the onions in the pan. Drizzle with the oil. Stir to coat. Spread the onions in a single layer.

Roast for 30 minutes, or until the onions begin to brown on the edges, stirring halfway through. Transfer to a small bowl.

Preheat the broiler. Lightly spray the broiler pan with cooking spray.

Stir ⅛ teaspoon salt, remaining 1 teaspoon chili garlic sauce or paste, and remaining 1 tablespoon brown sugar into the onions. Cover to keep warm.

½ cup dry red wine (regular or nonalcoholic)

1 tablespoon light brown sugar and 1 tablespoon light brown sugar, divided use

1 teaspoon chili garlic sauce or paste and 1 teaspoon chili garlic sauce or paste (lowest sodium available), divided use

1 1-pound boneless sirloin steak, all visible fat discarded

Cooking spray

2 large onions (about 8 ounces each), thinly sliced lengthwise

2 teaspoons canola or corn oil

⅛ teaspoon salt and ¼ teaspoon salt, divided use

Drain the beef, discarding the marinade. Sprinkle with the remaining ¼ teaspoon salt. Transfer to the broiler pan.

Broil the beef about 6 inches from the heat for 3 minutes on each side, or to the desired doneness. Transfer to a cutting board and let stand for 5 minutes. Slice the beef. Serve topped with the onion mixture.

PER SERVING

calories 216	**cholesterol** 56 mg	**protein** 25 g	**dietary exchanges**
total fat 6.5 g	**sodium** 280 mg	**calcium** 35 mg	2 vegetable
saturated 2.0 g	**carbohydrates** 13 g	**potassium** 455 mg	3 lean meat
trans 0.0 g	fiber 2 g		
polyunsaturated 1.0 g	sugars 9 g		
monounsaturated 3.5 g			

SIRLOIN with Tomato, Olive, and Feta Topping

This steak fits right into your schedule—it can marinate for as little as 30 minutes or as long as 8 hours—and it is equally good whether cooked on the stovetop, grilled, or broiled. Rice and Vegetable Pilaf (page 252) goes well with it.

SERVES 4 | 3 ounces beef and ½ cup topping per serving

In a large shallow glass dish, stir together the lemon zest, lemon juice, garlic, oregano, and pepper. Add the beef, turning to coat. Cover and refrigerate for 30 minutes to 8 hours, turning occasionally.

Meanwhile, in a medium bowl, stir together the topping ingredients. Cover and refrigerate until ready to serve.

Drain the beef, discarding the marinade.

Heat a large nonstick skillet over medium-high heat. Cook the beef for 4 to 5 minutes on each side, or to the desired doneness. (If you prefer, grill the beef on medium high or broil it 5 to 6 inches from the heat as directed.) Serve the beef with the topping.

SIRLOIN

- 1 teaspoon grated lemon zest
- 2 tablespoons fresh lemon juice
- 2 medium garlic cloves, minced
- 1 teaspoon dried oregano, crumbled
- ¼ teaspoon pepper
- 1 pound boneless top sirloin steak, all visible fat discarded, cut into 4 pieces

TOPPING

- 2 cups grape tomatoes or cherry tomatoes, halved
- 2 tablespoons chopped kalamata olives
- 2 tablespoons crumbled fat-free feta cheese
- 1 tablespoon red wine vinegar

PER SERVING

calories 179	**cholesterol** 56 mg	**protein** 26 g	**dietary exchanges**
total fat 5.5 g	**sodium** 186 mg	**calcium** 35 mg	1 vegetable
saturated 2.0 g	**carbohydrates** 6 g	**potassium** 542 mg	3 lean meat
trans 0.0 g	fiber 1 g		
polyunsaturated 0.5 g	sugars 3 g		
monounsaturated 3.0 g			

FILETS MIGNONS
with Brandy au Jus

Reducing the liquid for this dish yields an intensely flavored sauce, so a little is all you need.

SERVES 4 | 3 ounces beef and 1 tablespoon sauce per serving

Preheat the oven to 200°F.

In a small bowl, stir together the water, 2 tablespoons brandy, bouillon granules, and Worcestershire sauce. Set aside.

Lightly spray a large skillet with cooking spray. Heat over high heat. Sprinkle the salt over the beef. Cook the beef for 2 minutes on each side. Reduce the heat to medium. Cook for 2 to 6 minutes, or to the desired doneness. Transfer the beef to an ovenproof plate. Put in the oven to keep warm.

Return the skillet (don't drain) to the heat. Increase the heat to high. Pour the brandy mixture into the skillet, scraping the bottom and side to dislodge any browned bits. Bring to a boil. Boil for 4 minutes, or until the liquid is reduced to ¼ cup, stirring constantly. Remove from the heat.

Add the margarine and remaining ½ teaspoon brandy, stirring until the margarine has melted.

Transfer the beef to plates. Spoon the sauce over the beef. Sprinkle with the pepper and parsley.

¾ cup water

2 tablespoons brandy and ½ teaspoon brandy (optional), divided use

1 teaspoon very low sodium beef bouillon granules

1 teaspoon Worcestershire sauce (lowest sodium available)

Cooking spray

⅛ teaspoon salt

4 filets mignons (about 4 ounces each), all visible fat (and bacon, if any) discarded

1 teaspoon light tub margarine

¼ teaspoon pepper

2 tablespoons snipped fresh parsley

PER SERVING

calories 174	**cholesterol** 57 mg	**protein** 24 g	**dietary exchanges**
total fat 5.0 g	**sodium** 135 mg	**calcium** 9 mg	3 lean meat
saturated 2.5 g	**carbohydrates** 1 g	**potassium** 387 mg	
trans 0.0 g	fiber 0 g		
polyunsaturated 0.5 g	sugars 0 g		
monounsaturated 2.5 g			

PACIFIC RIM FLANK STEAK

Pineapple juice adds a taste of Hawaii to the slightly sweet yet spicy marinade in this dish, and chili garlic sauce adds a bit of Asian flair. Be sure to allow time to marinate the steak for 8 to 24 hours. The recipe makes enough for you to serve grilled steak tonight and have some left for Pacific Rim Steak Salad with Sweet-and-Sour Dressing (page 94) later in the week.

SERVES 4 | 3 ounces beef per serving (plus 8 ounces reserved)

In a medium glass dish, stir together the marinade ingredients. Add the beef, turning to coat. Cover and refrigerate for 8 to 24 hours, turning occasionally.

Preheat the broiler. Lightly spray a broiler pan and rack with cooking spray.

Remove the beef from the dish, discarding the marinade. Transfer the beef to the broiler rack.

Broil 4 to 6 inches from the heat for 3 to 7 minutes on each side, or to the desired doneness (3 to 5 minutes on each side for medium rare, 4 to 7 minutes on each side for medium). Transfer the beef to a cutting board. Cut diagonally across the grain into very thin slices.

MARINADE

¾ cup pineapple juice

¼ cup snipped fresh cilantro

2 tablespoons grated sweet onion, such as Vidalia, Maui, or Oso Sweet

2 teaspoons chili garlic sauce or paste (lowest sodium available)

2 teaspoons Worcestershire sauce (lowest sodium available)

1 teaspoon olive oil (extra virgin preferred)

2 medium garlic cloves, crushed

⅛ teaspoon pepper

1 1½-pound flank steak, all visible fat discarded

Cooking spray

COOK'S TIP If you plan to make the steak salad, you will see that it calls for pineapple chunks canned in their own juice. That juice is too mild for the steak marinade, which is why we don't use it in this recipe. Regular canned pineapple juice will provide considerably more flavor.

COOK'S TIP ON CHILI GARLIC SAUCE OR PASTE Chili garlic sauce is a deliciously spicy blend of coarsely ground chiles and garlic. It is interchangeable with chili garlic paste, which includes the same ingredients plus vinegar. Look for these products in the international section of most major supermarkets. Try adding them to a variety of foods, such as chicken, fish, beef, and pasta.

PER SERVING

calories 162	**cholesterol** 48 mg	**protein** 23 g	**dietary exchanges**
total fat 6.5 g	**sodium** 77 mg	**calcium** 4 mg	3 lean meat
saturated 3.0 g	**carbohydrates** 0 g	**potassium** 222 mg	
trans 0.0 g	fiber 0 g		
polyunsaturated 0.5 g	sugars 0 g		
monounsaturated 3.0 g			

GRILLED FLANK STEAK AND ASPARAGUS with Couscous

You'll need to plan ahead for this Mediterranean-Middle Eastern combo; the flank steak marinates for 6 to 8 hours. Since meat, vegetables, and grain are included in this dish, all you need to add is some sliced tomatoes or a light dessert.

SERVES 4 | 3 ounces beef, ½ cup vegetables, and ½ cup couscous per serving

Put the beef in a large shallow dish.

In a small bowl, stir together 2 tablespoons lemon juice, 1 minced garlic clove, and the pepper. Drizzle over the beef. Turn the beef to coat. Cover and refrigerate for 6 to 8 hours, turning once halfway through.

Lightly spray the grill rack with cooking spray. Preheat the grill on medium high.

In a small bowl, stir together the oil, basil, thyme, remaining ⅓ cup lemon juice, and remaining 2 minced garlic cloves.

Place the asparagus spears and bell pepper in a separate large shallow dish. Drizzle with 2 tablespoons of the oil mixture. Turn to coat.

Spoon 1 tablespoon of the remaining oil mixture into a cup. Set aside the oil mixture in the cup and the oil mixture still in the small bowl.

Drain the beef, discarding the marinade.

Grill the beef, covered, for about 20 minutes, or until the desired doneness, turning once halfway through and brushing frequently with the oil mixture from the bowl, using a clean brush each time. When the beef has grilled for about 10 minutes, put the bell pepper on the

- 1 **1-pound flank steak, all visible fat discarded**
- 2 **tablespoons fresh lemon juice and ⅓ cup fresh lemon juice, divided use**
- 1 **medium garlic clove, minced, and 2 medium garlic cloves, minced, divided use**
- ¼ **teaspoon pepper**
- **Cooking spray**
- 2 **teaspoons olive oil**
- 1 **teaspoon dried basil, crumbled**
- 1 **teaspoon dried thyme, crumbled**
- 12 **ounces thin asparagus spears (about 40; uniform size preferred), trimmed**
- 1 **medium red bell pepper, quartered**
- 1¼ **cups water**
- ¾ **cup uncooked whole-wheat couscous**

grill. About 5 minutes later, add the asparagus. Grill the bell pepper and asparagus until tender-crisp, turning and brushing frequently with the oil mixture.

Transfer the beef and bell pepper to separate cutting boards; transfer the asparagus to a medium plate. Cover the beef and let stand for 5 minutes. Slice the beef across the grain into thin strips. Slice the bell pepper into lengthwise strips.

Meanwhile, in a medium saucepan, bring the water just to a boil. Stir in the couscous. Remove from the heat and let stand, covered, for 5 minutes. Lightly fluff with a fork.

Drizzle with the reserved 1 tablespoon oil mixture from the cup. Spoon the couscous onto a serving platter. Arrange the beef, bell pepper, and asparagus on the couscous.

COOK'S TIP If you buy thicker asparagus spears, it may take up to 6 minutes of grilling time for them to become tender-crisp. Whether you buy thin or thick asparagus, try to get spears of uniform size so they will cook evenly.

PER SERVING

calories 376	cholesterol 37 mg	protein 33 g	dietary exchanges
total fat 9.5 g	sodium 69 mg	calcium 84 mg	2½ starch
saturated 3.0 g	carbohydrates 43 g	potassium 681 mg	1 vegetable
trans 0.0 g	fiber 8 g		3 lean meat
polyunsaturated 1.0 g	sugars 4 g		
monounsaturated 4.0 g			

MEAT LOAF

Yogurt in meat loaf? Plain yogurt not only provides potassium but also is a great way to keep meat loaf moist.

SERVES 8 | 2 slices per serving

Preheat the oven to 375°F. Lightly spray a 9-inch square baking pan with cooking spray. Set aside.

In a large bowl, stir together the oatmeal and yogurt. Let stand for 5 minutes.

Add the remaining ingredients. Combine using your hands or a spoon. Shape into a loaf about 8 x 5 inches. Place in the baking pan.

Bake for about 1 hour 15 minutes, or until the meat loaf registers 165°F on an instant-read thermometer and is no longer pink in the center. Remove from the oven and let stand for 5 to 10 minutes. Cut into 16 slices.

Cooking spray
- ½ cup uncooked quick-cooking oatmeal
- ¼ cup fat-free plain yogurt
- 1 pound extra-lean ground beef
- ½ cup chopped onion
- 1 medium rib of celery, chopped
- 1 small carrot or parsnip, shredded
- ¼ cup egg substitute or 1 large egg
- 1 tablespoon capers packed in balsamic vinegar, drained
- 1 tablespoon fresh lemon juice
- ½ teaspoon dried thyme, crumbled
- ¼ teaspoon pepper
- ¼ teaspoon garlic powder

COOK'S TIP For leftovers with style, make meat loaf sandwiches in low-sodium buns or on low-sodium bread. Top the meat loaf with a mixture of 1 tablespoon no-salt-added ketchup and ½ teaspoon bottled white horseradish or dried horse-radish. Add some crunchy romaine or curly green leaf lettuce, sliced onion, and Easy Dill Pickles (page 272). For a different flavor, spread the meat loaf with Barbecue Sauce (page 265) or Roasted Tomato Chipotle Salsa (page 269).

PER SERVING

calories 119	cholesterol 31 mg	protein 15 g	**dietary exchanges**
total fat 3.0 g	**sodium** 102 mg	**calcium** 33 mg	½ starch
saturated 1.0 g	**carbohydrates** 8 g	**potassium** 248 mg	2 very lean meat
trans 0.0 g	fiber 2 g		
polyunsaturated 0.5 g	sugars 2 g		
monounsaturated 1.5 g			

BEEF AND PORTOBELLO PASTA

Portobello mushrooms have a meaty texture that's perfect for this classic meat-lovers' dish.

SERVES 4 | 1 cup per serving

Prepare the pasta using the package directions, omitting the salt. Drain well in a colander. Set aside.

Meanwhile, in a large nonstick saucepan, cook the beef, mushroom, onion, and garlic over medium-high heat for 8 to 10 minutes, or until the beef is browned on the outside and the mushroom and onion are soft, stirring occasionally to turn and break up the beef. Drain if necessary. Wipe the skillet with paper towels. Return the drained mixture to the skillet.

Stir in the remaining ingredients. Bring to a simmer over medium-high heat. Reduce the heat to medium low and cook for 15 minutes, stirring occasionally.

Stir in the pasta. Cook for 2 to 3 minutes, or until heated through. Discard the bay leaf before serving the dish.

1 cup dried whole-grain small shell macaroni

1 pound extra-lean ground beef

1 medium portobello mushroom, stem trimmed, cut into ¾-inch cubes (about 1 cup)

1 cup chopped onion

1 medium garlic clove, minced

1 14.5-ounce can no-salt-added diced tomatoes, undrained

1 8-ounce can no-salt-added tomato sauce

½ cup water

1 medium dried bay leaf

1 teaspoon sugar

1 teaspoon dried Italian seasoning, crumbled

½ teaspoon pepper

½ teaspoon crushed red pepper flakes (optional)

PER SERVING

calories 309	**cholesterol** 62 mg	**protein** 31 g	**dietary exchanges**
total fat 6.5 g	**sodium** 108 mg	**calcium** 66 mg	1½ starch
saturated 2.5 g	**carbohydrates** 35 g	**potassium** 855 mg	3 vegetable
trans 0.5 g	fiber 5 g		3 lean meat
polyunsaturated 1.0 g	sugars 8 g		
monounsaturated 2.5 g			

SPAGHETTI
with Meat Sauce

When you want to serve a crowd but don't want to spend all day in the kitchen, this great recipe is the answer.

SERVES 12 | 1 cup spaghetti and ⅔ cup sauce per serving

In a large saucepan, cook the beef over medium-high heat for 3 to 4 minutes, or until browned on the outside and no longer pink in the center, stirring frequently to turn and break up the beef. Drain if necessary. Wipe the pan with paper towels. Return the beef to the pan.

Stir in the remaining ingredients except the pasta. Simmer, covered, for 1 hour 30 minutes, stirring occasionally. If the sauce seems too thick, gradually add water until the desired consistency.

Meanwhile, prepare the pasta using the package directions, omitting the salt. Drain well in a colander. Serve topped with the sauce.

- 1 pound extra-lean ground beef
- 1 28-ounce can no-salt-added diced tomatoes, undrained
- 2 small zucchini, diced
- 1 6-ounce can no-salt-added tomato paste
- 1 medium onion, chopped
- ½ cup dry red wine (regular or nonalcoholic)
- 1½ teaspoons chopped fresh oregano or ½ teaspoon dried, crumbled
- 1½ teaspoons chopped fresh basil or ½ teaspoon dried, crumbled
- 1 medium garlic clove, minced
- ½ teaspoon fennel seeds
- ⅛ teaspoon pepper
- 24 ounces dried whole-grain spaghetti

PER SERVING

calories 287
total fat 3.0 g
  saturated 1.0 g
  trans 0.0 g
  polyunsaturated 0.5 g
  monounsaturated 1.0 g

cholesterol 21 mg
sodium 57 mg
carbohydrates 50 g
  fiber 9 g
  sugars 7 g

protein 18 g
calcium 58 mg
potassium 575 mg

dietary exchanges
  3 starch
  1 vegetable
  1 very lean meat

SLOW-COOKER BEEF AND RED BEANS

With cayenne for a bit of kick and imitation bacon bits for smoky flavor, this hearty combination of ground beef, red beans, brown rice, and vegetables is sure to be a family-pleaser.

SERVES 6 | 1 cup beef mixture and ½ cup rice per serving

In a large skillet, cook the beef over medium-high heat for 7 to 8 minutes, or until browned on the outside and no longer pink in the center, stirring frequently to turn and break up the beef. Using a slotted spoon, transfer the beef to a 3½- or 4-quart slow cooker.

Stir in the broth, beans, tomatoes with liquid, 1 cup water, the celery, onion, bell pepper, bacon bits, thyme, garlic, pepper, and cayenne. Cook, covered, on high for 3 to 4 hours or on low for 7 to 8 hours.

Prepare the rice using the remaining 1⅔ cups water (this may differ from the package directions) and the seasoning blend, omitting the salt and margarine. Serve topped with the beef mixture.

- 1 pound extra-lean ground beef
- 2 cups Chicken Broth (page 50) or commercial fat-free, low-sodium chicken broth
- 1 15.5-ounce can no-salt-added red beans, rinsed and drained
- 1 14.5-ounce can no-salt-added diced tomatoes, undrained
- 1 cup water and 1⅔ cups water, divided use
- 2 medium ribs of celery, chopped
- ½ medium onion, chopped
- ½ medium green bell pepper, chopped
- 2 tablespoons imitation bacon bits
- 1 teaspoon dried thyme, crumbled
- 2 medium garlic cloves, minced

(continued)

COOK'S TIP If you prefer to cook the rice in the slow cooker, stir it in 30 minutes before the end of the cooking time (on high or low setting). If using this method, be sure to add the 1⅔ cups water and the seasoning blend to the slow cooker when you add the beef, beans, and vegetables. You'll save on washing an extra pan, but the presentation won't be quite as attractive.

¼ teaspoon pepper

⅛ to ¼ teaspoon cayenne

1½ cups uncooked instant brown rice

1 teaspoon salt-free all-purpose seasoning blend

PER SERVING

calories 275	**cholesterol** 42 mg	**protein** 24 g	**dietary exchanges**
total fat 5.5 g	**sodium** 156 mg	**calcium** 65 mg	2 starch
saturated 1.5 g	**carbohydrates** 33 g	**potassium** 596 mg	1 vegetable
trans 0.0 g	fiber 5 g		2½ lean meat
polyunsaturated 0.5 g	sugars 3 g		
monounsaturated 2.0 g			

CHILI

Before or after the football game, a "bowl of red" is a sure winner.

SERVES 4 | 1 cup per serving

In a Dutch oven, cook the beef over high heat for 3 to 4 minutes, or until browned on the outside and no longer pink in the center, stirring frequently to turn and break up the beef. Drain if necessary. Wipe the pot with paper towels. Return the beef to the pot.

Reduce the heat to medium-high. Stir in the onion and jalapeño. Cook for 3 minutes, or until the onion is soft, stirring frequently.

Stir in the remaining ingredients. Reduce the heat and simmer, covered, for 1 hour 30 minutes, stirring occasionally. Add water as needed for the desired consistency.

COOK'S TIP ON CHILI POWDER Our homemade no-salt-added variety (page 277) provides the flavor without the sodium. If you're using commercial chili powder instead, be sure to check labels. Most bottled chili powder contains salt, so look for the brand with the least amount. Or, in a pinch, substitute a mixture of 2 parts paprika to 1 part ground cumin.

1 pound extra-lean ground beef

½ cup chopped onion

1 to 2 tablespoons chopped fresh jalapeño

1 15.5-ounce can no-salt-added pinto beans, undrained

1 14.5-ounce can no-salt-added stewed tomatoes, undrained

½ cup water (plus more as needed)

¼ cup stout or beer (regular, light, or nonalcoholic)

1 tablespoon Chili Powder (page 277) or no-salt-added chili powder

2 teaspoons ground cumin

½ teaspoon dried oregano, crumbled

¼ teaspoon garlic powder

¼ teaspoon salt

⅛ teaspoon pepper

⅛ teaspoon cayenne (optional)

PER SERVING

calories 300	**cholesterol** 62 mg	**protein** 32 g	**dietary exchanges**
total fat 6.0 g	**sodium** 249 mg	**calcium** 95 mg	1 starch
saturated 2.5 g	**carbohydrates** 28 g	**potassium** 706 mg	2 vegetable
trans 0.5 g	fiber 7 g		3½ lean meat
polyunsaturated 0.5 g	sugars 9 g		
monounsaturated 2.5 g			

ONE-SKILLET BEEF, PASTA, AND BROCCOLI

Give leftover beef (or pork) a well-balanced makeover by adding bell pepper, broccoli, and whole-grain pasta. The result is an easy one-skillet meal.

SERVES 4 | 1½ cups per serving

In a large skillet, heat the oil over medium heat, swirling to coat the bottom. Cook the bell pepper and onion for 3 to 4 minutes, or until tender, stirring occasionally.

Stir in the broth, beef, Worcestershire sauce, savory, and pepper. Increase the heat to medium high and bring to a simmer.

Stir in the pasta. Reduce the heat and simmer, covered, for 5 minutes.

Stir in the broccoli. Simmer, covered, for 5 minutes, or until the pasta and broccoli are tender.

- 1 teaspoon olive oil
- 1 medium bell pepper (any color), thinly sliced
- 1 medium onion, thinly sliced
- 2 cups Beef Broth (page 52) or commercial fat-free, no-salt-added beef broth
- 12 ounces cubed cooked lean beef or pork roast, cooked without salt, all visible fat discarded
- 2 teaspoons Worcestershire sauce (lowest sodium available)
- 1 teaspoon dried savory or dried oregano, crumbled
- ¼ teaspoon pepper
- 4 ounces dried whole-grain pasta, such as rotelle or macaroni
- 3 ounces broccoli florets

COOK'S TIP ON SAVORY This interesting herb is worth experimenting with. A member of the mint family, it is slightly peppery. The two most popular varieties are summer savory, which is more delicate, and winter savory, which is spicier and sharper; they are interchangeable. Try savory in bean, pea, and lentil dishes (it is called the bean herb in continental Europe), as well as in stews, marinades, soups, salads, and more.

PER SERVING

calories 286
total fat 4.0 g
  saturated 1.5 g
  trans 0.0 g
  polyunsaturated 0.5 g
  monounsaturated 2.0 g

cholesterol 55 mg
sodium 76 mg
carbohydrates 28 g
  fiber 6 g
  sugars 5 g

protein 35 g
calcium 50 mg
potassium 557 mg

dietary exchanges
1½ starch
1 vegetable
3 very lean meat

DIJON PORK TENDERLOIN
with Marmalade Rice

While the pork roasts in its herb-enhanced Dijon glaze, you can prepare the brown rice flavored with orange marmalade that accompanies it. Steam some broccoli to serve on the side.

SERVES 4 | 3 ounces pork and ½ cup rice per serving

Preheat the oven to 350°F.

In a small bowl, stir together the mustard, rosemary, oregano, vinegar, and pepper. Using a pastry brush or spoon, brush over the pork. Transfer the pork to an 8-inch square nonstick baking dish.

Roast for 40 to 45 minutes, or until the pork registers 150°F on an instant-read thermometer, or is slightly pink in the very center. Remove from the oven and let the pork stand in the baking dish for about 10 minutes to continue cooking. It will reach about 160°F. Slice the pork crosswise.

When you remove the pork from the oven, put the broth and marmalade in a medium saucepan and bring to a boil over high heat. Stir in the rice. Reduce the heat and simmer, covered, for 10 minutes, or until the liquid is absorbed and the rice is tender. Serve the pork slices on the rice.

2 tablespoons Dijon mustard (lowest sodium available)

1 tablespoon chopped fresh rosemary or 1 teaspoon dried, crushed

1 tablespoon chopped fresh oregano or 1 teaspoon dried, crumbled

2 teaspoons cider vinegar

¼ teaspoon pepper

1 1-pound pork tenderloin, all visible fat discarded

1¼ cups Chicken Broth (page 50) or commercial fat-free, low-sodium chicken broth

2 tablespoons all-fruit orange marmalade

1 cup uncooked instant brown rice

PER SERVING

calories 270	**cholesterol** 75 mg	**protein** 28 g	**dietary exchanges**
total fat 6.5 g	**sodium** 219 mg	**calcium** 18 mg	1 starch
saturated 2.0 g	**carbohydrates** 24 g	**potassium** 438 mg	½ fruit
trans 0.0 g	fiber 1 g		3 lean meat
polyunsaturated 1.0 g	sugars 5 g		
monounsaturated 2.5 g			

HUNGARIAN PORK CHOPS

An Old World comfort dish without the work, these pork chops pair nicely with whole-grain noodles and steamed brussels sprouts.

SERVES 4 | 3 ounces pork and 3 tablespoons sauce per serving

In a small bowl, stir together the rub ingredients. Sprinkle on both sides of the pork. Using your fingertips, gently press the rub so it adheres to the pork.

Lightly spray a large, heavy skillet with cooking spray. Heat over medium-high heat. Reduce the heat to medium. Cook the pork for 4 minutes. Turn over and cook for 4 to 5 minutes, or until slightly pink in the center. Transfer to a large plate. Cover to keep warm.

Increase the heat to high. Pour in the water, scraping the skillet to dislodge any browned bits. Boil for 1 to 2 minutes, or until the liquid is reduced to ¼ cup. Reduce the heat to low.

When the boiling stops, whisk in the sour cream and salt. Cook for 2 to 3 minutes, or until heated through, whisking constantly. Don't let the mixture boil. Serve the sauce over the pork. Sprinkle the green onion on top.

RUB

- 1 teaspoon paprika
- ¾ teaspoon dried dillweed, crumbled
- ½ teaspoon caraway seeds
- ½ teaspoon onion powder
- ½ teaspoon garlic powder

- 4 boneless center loin pork chops (about 4 ounces each), cut ½ inch thick, all visible fat discarded
- Cooking spray
- ½ cup water
- ½ cup fat-free sour cream
- ¼ teaspoon salt
- 2 tablespoons finely chopped green onion

PER SERVING

calories 196	**cholesterol** 72 mg	**protein** 26 g	**dietary exchanges**
total fat 6.5 g	**sodium** 222 mg	**calcium** 87 mg	½ other carbohydrate
saturated 2.5 g	**carbohydrates** 7 g	**potassium** 404 mg	3 lean meat
trans 0.0 g	fiber 1 g		
polyunsaturated 0.5 g	sugars 3 g		
monounsaturated 3.0 g			

CARIBBEAN JERK PORK

Enjoy a delicious island meal by making your own fragrant jerk seasoning to flavor grilled or broiled pork chops.

SERVES 4 | 3 ounces pork per serving

Lightly spray the grill rack or broiler pan and rack with cooking spray. Preheat the grill on high or preheat the broiler.

In a food processor or blender, process all the seasoning blend ingredients until smooth. Transfer to a large shallow glass dish.

Add the pork to the seasoning blend, turning to coat. Cover and refrigerate for 15 to 20 minutes, turning occasionally.

Grill the pork or broil about 4 inches from the heat for 5 to 6 minutes on each side, or until slightly pink in the center. Sprinkle with the salt. Serve with the lime wedges to squeeze on top.

Cooking spray

SEASONING BLEND

1 or 2 medium fresh jalapeños, halved lengthwise, stem(s), ribs, and seeds discarded

2 tablespoons chopped onion

1 tablespoon ground allspice

1 tablespoon chopped fresh thyme or 1 teaspoon dried, crumbled

1 teaspoon grated orange zest

2 tablespoons fresh orange juice

1 tablespoon honey

2 teaspoons steak sauce (lowest sodium available)

½ teaspoon ground cinnamon

---

4 boneless center loin pork chops (about 4 ounces each), all visible fat discarded

¼ teaspoon salt

1 medium lime, cut into 4 wedges (optional)

COOK'S TIP ON JERKING AND JERK SEASONING Jerking, a method of cooking in Jamaica, involves rubbing meat with, or marinating it in, a fiery-hot, intensely flavored mixture, then grilling it. Although chicken and pork are the most commonly jerked foods, beef, goat, and fish can also be prepared this way. Jerk seasoning almost always includes some Scotch bonnet or habanero chiles, but we lowered the heat a notch here by using jalapeño. Other very typical jerk seasonings are allspice, cinnamon, ginger, nutmeg, cloves, thyme, garlic, and onions.

PER SERVING

calories 173
total fat 6.0 g
  saturated 2.0 g
  trans 0.0 g
  polyunsaturated 0.5 g
  monounsaturated 2.0 g

cholesterol 66 mg
sodium 229 mg
carbohydrates 8 g
  fiber 1 g
  sugars 5 g

protein 22 g
calcium 42 mg
potassium 349 mg

dietary exchanges
½ other carbohydrate
3 lean meat

PORK CHOPS
with Herb Rub

Marjoram, an aromatic herb that tastes like a mild version of oregano, is the key ingredient in the rub that makes these grilled pork chops so tasty.

SERVES 4 | 3 ounces pork per serving

Preheat the grill on medium high or preheat the broiler.

In a small bowl, stir together all the ingredients except the pork. Sprinkle over both sides of the pork. Using your fingertips, gently press the mixture so it adheres to the pork.

Grill the pork or broil about 4 inches from the heat for 5 to 6 minutes on each side, or until browned on the outside and slightly pink in the center.

½ teaspoon dried marjoram, crumbled

⅛ teaspoon garlic powder

⅛ teaspoon onion powder

⅛ teaspoon pepper

4 center loin pork chops (about 4 ounces each if boneless, 6 ounces each with bone), cut ½ inch thick, all visible fat discarded

PER SERVING

calories 143
total fat 6.0 g
  saturated 1.5 g
  trans 0.0 g
  polyunsaturated 0.5 g
  monounsaturated 2.0 g

cholesterol 66 mg
sodium 44 mg
carbohydrates 0 g
  fiber 0 g
  sugars 0 g

protein 21 g
calcium 20 mg
potassium 285 mg

dietary exchanges
3 lean meat

BAKED PORK CHOPS
with Apple Dressing

No more dry pork chops! Just "sandwich" the chops between layers of dressing and bake, leaving them tender and moist. Serve with green beans tossed with lemon zest.

SERVES 4 | 3 ounces meat and ½ cup dressing per serving

Preheat the oven to 375°F.

In a medium bowl, stir together the dressing ingredients until the bread is moistened. Spoon half the dressing into an 8-inch square baking pan, smoothing the surface. Place the pork in a single layer on the dressing. Spread the remaining dressing over the pork.

Bake, covered, for 30 minutes. Uncover and bake for about 10 minutes, or until the pork is slightly pink in the center and the dressing is golden brown. Using a wide spatula, transfer the dressing-covered pork to plates. Spoon any remaining dressing over the pork.

DRESSING

- 2 slices light whole-wheat bread (lowest sodium available), torn into bite-size pieces
- 1 medium apple, such as Granny Smith, Gala, Fuji, or Golden Delicious, peeled and finely chopped
- 1 medium rib of celery, finely chopped
- 4 medium green onions (green and white parts), thinly sliced
- ¼ cup Chicken Broth (page 50) or commercial fat-free, low-sodium chicken broth
- ¼ cup egg substitute or 1 large egg
- 1 teaspoon dried sage
- ¼ teaspoon pepper

- 4 boneless center loin pork chops (about 4 ounces each), all visible fat discarded

PER SERVING

calories 238	**cholesterol** 66 mg	**protein** 26 g	**dietary exchanges**
total fat 6.5 g	**sodium** 221 mg	**calcium** 60 mg	½ starch
saturated 2.0 g	**carbohydrates** 18 g	**potassium** 507 mg	½ fruit
trans 0.0 g	fiber 5 g		3 lean meat
polyunsaturated 1.0 g	sugars 6 g		
monounsaturated 2.5 g			

LAMB CURRY

Serve this spicy lamb over whole-wheat couscous with small bowls of raisins and sliced green onions to sprinkle on top.

SERVES 8 | 3 ounces lamb per serving

In a medium shallow dish, stir together the flour and pepper. Add the lamb, a few pieces at a time, turning to coat and gently shaking off any excess.

In a large nonstick skillet, heat the oil over medium-high heat, swirling to coat the bottom. Cook the lamb for about 5 minutes, or until browned on all sides, stirring occasionally. Using a slotted spoon, transfer the lamb to a plate. Pour off the excess fat. Wipe the skillet clean with paper towels. Return the lamb to the skillet.

Stir in the remaining ingredients except the lemon juice. Simmer, covered, for 1 hour, or until the lamb is tender, stirring occasionally.

Just before serving, stir in the lemon juice.

3 tablespoons all-purpose flour

⅛ teaspoon pepper

2 pounds boneless lamb chuck roast, all visible fat discarded, cut into cubes

2 teaspoons canola or corn oil

3 cups water

½ cup finely chopped onion

½ cup unsweetened applesauce

2 to 3 teaspoons curry powder

2 teaspoons fresh lemon juice

PER SERVING

calories 175	**cholesterol** 65 mg	**protein** 20 g	**dietary exchanges**
total fat 7.5 g	**sodium** 62 mg	**calcium** 21 mg	½ other carbohydrate
saturated 2.5 g	**carbohydrates** 5 g	**potassium** 282 mg	3 lean meat
trans 0.0 g	fiber 1 g		
polyunsaturated 1.0 g	sugars 2 g		
monounsaturated 3.5 g			

VEGETARIAN ENTRÉES

THREE-CHEESE LASAGNA
with Swiss Chard

Layers of cheese, chunky tomatoes, and earthy greens make this one of the best vegetarian lasagnas you'll try.

SERVES 6 | 2½ x 4-inch square per serving

In a large saucepan, combine the chard and water. Bring to a boil over high heat. Reduce the heat and simmer, covered, for 5 minutes, or until tender. Drain well in a colander. Let cool for about 10 minutes, or until easy to handle. Squeeze the chard dry. Transfer to a medium bowl.

Meanwhile, cook the pasta using the package directions, omitting the salt. Don't overcook. Drain well in a colander. Cut a long piece of wax paper. Place the noodles in a single layer on the wax paper. Using paper towels, pat the noodles dry. Set aside.

Preheat the oven to 375°F. Lightly spray an 8-inch square glass baking dish and a piece of aluminum foil large enough to cover the dish with cooking spray. Set the dish and foil aside.

Heat the oil in a medium nonstick skillet over medium-high heat, swirling to coat the bottom. Cook the onion for 2 minutes, or until almost soft, stirring frequently.

Stir in the garlic. Cook for 1 minute, stirring constantly.

1   14- to 16-ounce bunch red or green Swiss chard, stems discarded, leaves chopped (about 8 cups)
1   cup water
9   dried whole-grain lasagna noodles

Cooking spray

2   teaspoons olive oil
1   medium onion, diced
2   medium garlic cloves, minced
2   14.5-ounce cans no-salt-added diced tomatoes, well drained
½   teaspoon dried basil, crumbled
⅛   teaspoon pepper and ⅛ teaspoon pepper, divided use
1   cup shredded low-fat mozzarella cheese
1   cup fat-free ricotta cheese
2   tablespoons shredded or grated Parmesan cheese

Stir in the tomatoes, basil, and ⅛ teaspoon pepper. Bring to a boil. Reduce the heat and simmer for 5 minutes, or until the tomatoes are very soft, stirring occasionally.

Stir the mozzarella, ricotta, and remaining ⅛ teaspoon pepper into the chard.

Layer as follows in the baking dish: ½ cup tomato mixture; 3 noodles, trimmed to fit the dish; half the cheese mixture; ¾ cup tomato mixture; 3 noodles, trimmed; remaining cheese mixture; remaining tomato mixture; and final 3 noodles, trimmed. Cover tightly with the aluminum foil with the sprayed side down.

Bake for 25 minutes, or until the casserole is heated through. Sprinkle with the Parmesan. Bake, uncovered, for 5 minutes, or until the Parmesan melts. Let stand for 10 minutes to make cutting easier. Cut into 6 pieces. Using a wide spatula, transfer the pieces to plates.

COOK'S TIP Chard with dark green leaves and red stems (red chard) may be more strongly flavored than chard that is lighter in color. Either works well in this recipe.

PER SERVING

calories 287	**cholesterol** 18 mg	**protein** 17 g	**dietary exchanges**
total fat 6.5 g	**sodium** 380 mg	**calcium** 325 mg	2 starch
saturated 2.0 g	**carbohydrates** 40 g	**potassium** 749 mg	2 vegetable
trans 0.0 g	fiber 9 g		1½ lean meat
polyunsaturated 0.5 g	sugars 9 g		
monounsaturated 2.5 g			

ALFREDO LASAGNA
with Broccoli and Cauliflower

A creamy Alfredo-type sauce binds layers of pasta, vegetables, and cheeses in this vegetarian lasagna. No tomatoes allowed!

SERVES 8 | ¾ to 1 cup per serving

Preheat the oven to 375°F. Lightly spray a 2-quart casserole dish with cooking spray. Set aside.

In a medium saucepan, whisk together the sauce ingredients except the Parmesan. Cook over medium-high heat for 4 to 5 minutes, or until the mixture thickens slightly (it will still be somewhat thin), stirring occasionally.

Stir in the Parmesan. Remove from the heat. Set aside.

In a medium bowl, stir together the ricotta, egg substitute, oregano, onion powder, and garlic powder. Set aside.

If using fresh cauliflower and broccoli, in a medium saucepan, bring the water to a boil over high heat. Reduce the heat to medium high and cook the cauliflower for 2 minutes. Stir in the broccoli. Cook for 1 minute. Transfer to a colander. Drain well.

Cooking spray

SAUCE

2½ cups fat-free milk

3 tablespoons all-purpose flour

¼ teaspoon pepper

⅛ teaspoon cayenne (optional)

¼ cup shredded or grated Parmesan cheese

---

1 cup fat-free ricotta cheese

¼ cup egg substitute or 1 large egg

1 teaspoon dried oregano, crumbled

¼ teaspoon onion powder

¼ teaspoon garlic powder

4 cups water (if using fresh vegetables)

2 cups chopped fresh (½-inch pieces) or frozen cauliflower, thawed if frozen

(continued)

Layer as follows in the casserole dish: half the sauce, 4 noodle halves, all the ricotta mixture, and the cauliflower and broccoli. Sprinkle with the roasted pepper and ½ cup mozzarella. Top with the remaining noodle halves, remaining sauce, and remaining ½ cup mozzarella. Cover the dish and place on a baking sheet in case the lasagna bubbles over.

Bake for 30 minutes.

Meanwhile, in a small bowl, stir together the topping ingredients. When the lasagna has baked for 30 minutes, sprinkle with the topping. Bake, uncovered, for 8 to 10 minutes, or until the topping is toasted and the noodles are tender. Remove from the oven and let stand for 5 to 10 minutes to make cutting easier.

2 cups chopped fresh (½-inch pieces) or frozen broccoli, thawed if frozen

4 oven-ready lasagna noodles, broken in half crosswise

¼ cup roasted red bell pepper, chopped

½ cup shredded low-fat mozzarella cheese and ½ cup shredded low-fat mozzarella cheese, divided use

TOPPING

¼ cup plain dry bread crumbs (lowest sodium available)

2 teaspoons olive oil

½ teaspoon dried Italian seasoning, crumbled

PER SERVING

calories 184	**cholesterol** 15 mg	**protein** 15 g	**dietary exchanges**
total fat 4.5 g	**sodium** 278 mg	**calcium** 392 mg	1 starch
saturated 2.0 g	**carbohydrates** 20 g	**potassium** 377 mg	1 vegetable
trans 0.0 g	fiber 2 g		1½ lean meat
polyunsaturated 0.5 g	sugars 7 g		
monounsaturated 1.5 g			

FETTUCCINE ALFREDO

Now you can have all the richness of Alfredo sauce with only a fraction of the usual sodium, saturated fat, and calories. The addition of lemon gives this dish a fresh twist.

SERVES 8 | 1 cup per serving

Prepare the pasta using the package directions, omitting the salt. Drain well in a colander. Cover to keep warm.

Meanwhile, in a small bowl, whisk together ¼ cup milk and the flour until smooth. Heat a medium saucepan over medium heat. Pour the mixture into the saucepan.

Whisk in the remaining 1¼ cups milk. Bring to a boil. Cook for 15 minutes, or until thickened, stirring constantly with a flat spatula to keep the sauce from sticking to the bottom of the pan.

Stir in ¼ cup Parmesan and the lemon juice and pepper.

Transfer the pasta to a platter. Pour the sauce over the pasta. Sprinkle with the parsley, salt, and remaining 1½ tablespoons Parmesan. Garnish with the lemon wedges.

16 ounces dried whole-grain fettuccine

¼ cup fat-free milk and 1¼ cups fat-free milk, divided use

2 tablespoons all-purpose flour

¼ cup shredded or grated Parmesan cheese and 1½ tablespoons shredded or grated Parmesan cheese, divided use

2 teaspoons fresh lemon juice

⅛ teaspoon pepper (white preferred)

2 tablespoons finely snipped fresh parsley

¼ teaspoon salt

1 medium lemon, cut into 4 wedges (optional)

PER SERVING

calories 235	**cholesterol** 3 mg	**protein** 11 g	**dietary exchanges**
total fat 2.0 g	**sodium** 155 mg	**calcium** 125 mg	3 starch
saturated 1.0 g	**carbohydrates** 47 g	**potassium** 206 mg	½ very lean meat
trans 0.0 g	fiber 7 g		
polyunsaturated 0.5 g	sugars 4 g		
monounsaturated 0.5 g			

SPAGHETTI
with Fresh Mushroom Sauce

Use your own favorite mushroom variety, whatever the produce market is featuring this week, or a mixture to jazz up spaghetti with marinara sauce.

SERVES 4 | 1 cup spaghetti and ½ cup sauce per serving

In a large nonstick skillet, heat the oil over medium-high heat, swirling to coat the bottom. Cook the mushrooms, onion, and garlic for 3 to 5 minutes, or until the onion is soft, stirring occasionally.

Stir in the remaining ingredients except the pasta. Bring to a simmer. Reduce the heat and simmer, covered, for 1 to 2 hours, stirring occasionally. If the sauce becomes too thick, stir in a small amount of water. Discard the bay leaf.

Prepare the pasta using the package directions, omitting the salt. Drain well in a colander. Serve topped with the sauce.

1 tablespoon olive oil

1 cup sliced mushrooms, such as shiitake, brown (cremini), or portobello, or a combination

⅓ cup chopped onion

1 medium garlic clove, minced

1 14.5-ounce can no-salt-added diced tomatoes, undrained

1 6-ounce can no-salt-added tomato paste

½ cup water

1 tablespoon sugar

1 medium dried bay leaf

¾ teaspoon chopped fresh basil or ¼ teaspoon dried, crumbled

¾ teaspoon chopped fresh oregano or ¼ teaspoon dried, crumbled

⅛ teaspoon pepper

⅛ teaspoon cayenne (optional)

8 ounces dried whole-grain spaghetti

PER SERVING

calories 305	**cholesterol** 0 mg	**protein** 12 g	**dietary exchanges**
total fat 4.5 g	**sodium** 59 mg	**calcium** 77 mg	3 starch
saturated 0.5 g	**carbohydrates** 61 g	**potassium** 877 mg	3 vegetable
trans 0.0 g	fiber 10 g		
polyunsaturated 1.0 g	sugars 14 g		
monounsaturated 2.5 g			

FARRO RISOTTO
with Squash, Peas, and Feta

Crisply cooked yellow summer squash, green peas, and onion play deliciously off farro's earthy flavor.

SERVES 4 | 1½ cups per serving

In a large saucepan, heat the broth over medium-high heat for 8 to 10 minutes, or until hot. Reduce the heat to low to keep the broth hot.

Meanwhile, in another large saucepan, heat the oil over medium-high heat, swirling to coat the bottom. Cook the onion for 3 minutes, or until soft, stirring frequently.

Stir the farro into the onion. Ladle ½ cup broth into the mixture. Cook for 1 to 2 minutes, or until the broth is absorbed, stirring occasionally. Repeat the procedure, adding the remaining broth, ½ cup at a time, stirring until the broth is absorbed after each addition, about 5 minutes (the timing may vary from addition to addition). Stir in the squash and peas after 30 minutes of cooking time. (The total cooking time will be about 35 minutes.) Remove from the heat. Stir in the feta, dillweed, and lemon juice. Serve immediately so the farro doesn't become gummy.

4 cups Vegetable Broth (page 53) or commercial low-sodium vegetable broth

2 teaspoons olive oil

1 small onion, diced

1 cup uncooked farro

2 small yellow summer squash (about 6 ounces each), cut into ½-inch cubes

1 cup frozen green peas

½ cup crumbled low-fat feta cheese

2 tablespoons snipped fresh dillweed or ½ teaspoon dried dillweed, crumbled

1 tablespoon fresh lemon juice

COOK'S TIP You can use pearl barley instead of the farro in this recipe, but you will need to add about ½ cup water to the broth. The cooking time will be about the same.

COOK'S TIP ON FARRO An ancient grain grown for thousands of years in Italy and still often used in Italian cooking, farro is high in fiber and contains significantly more protein, but less gluten, than wheat. Farro looks much like light brown rice and has a nutty flavor and a chewy texture. Use it as a whole grain in dishes from soups to desserts or try ground farro as a substitute for wheat flour in pasta, pancakes, waffles, and baked goods.

PER SERVING

calories 271
total fat 4.0 g
  saturated 1.5 g
  trans 0.0 g
  polyunsaturated 0.5 g
  monounsaturated 2.0 g

cholesterol 5 mg
sodium 279 mg
carbohydrates 44 g
  fiber 6 g
  sugars 5 g

protein 13 g
calcium 28 mg
potassium 285 mg

dietary exchanges
2½ starch
1 vegetable
½ fat

TEX-MEX GRILLED VEGETABLES with Barley

Vegetables get plenty of smoky flavor when you grill them, so there's no need to reach for the salt shaker. Feel free to pop some other vegetables, such as yellow squash and mushrooms, onto the grill, too.

SERVES 4 | 1½ cups per serving

In a medium saucepan, bring the water to a boil over high heat. Stir in the barley. Reduce the heat and simmer, covered, for 10 to 12 minutes, or until the barley is tender and the water is absorbed. Set aside, still covered, to keep warm.

Lightly spray the grill rack with cooking spray. Preheat the grill on medium high.

In a small bowl, stir together the lime juice, cilantro, oil, garlic, cumin, and pepper. Spoon 1 tablespoon of the mixture into another small bowl. Set both bowls aside.

Arrange the onion, corn, bell peppers, zucchini, and jalapeño in a single layer on the grill.

Grill, covered, for 10 to 12 minutes, or until tender-crisp, turning as needed to cook evenly and brushing frequently with the larger amount of the lime juice mixture. As the vegetables become ready, transfer them to a rimmed baking sheet. Cover to keep warm.

2 cups water

1 cup uncooked quick-cooking barley

Cooking spray

¼ cup fresh lime juice

2 tablespoons snipped fresh cilantro

1 tablespoon olive oil

1 medium garlic clove, minced

½ teaspoon ground cumin

¼ teaspoon pepper

½ large sweet onion, such as Vidalia, Maui, or Oso Sweet, cut crosswise into ½-inch slices

1 medium ear of corn, silks and husks discarded

1 medium red bell pepper, quartered

1 medium green bell pepper, quartered

1 small to medium zucchini, cut lengthwise into quarters

(continued)

Remove the corn and jalapeño from the baking sheet. Cut the corn from the cob. Dice the jalapeño. Stir into the barley. Spoon onto a deep platter.

Remove the bell peppers, onion, and zucchini from the baking sheet. Cut the bell peppers into strips about 1 inch wide. Divide the onion slices into rings. Cut the zucchini pieces in half crosswise. Arrange the bell peppers, onion, and zucchini over the barley mixture. Drizzle with the reserved 1 tablespoon lime juice mixture. Sprinkle with the Mexican blend cheese.

1 medium fresh jalapeño, halved lengthwise, seeds and ribs discarded

2 tablespoons shredded low-fat 4-cheese Mexican blend or low-fat Monterey Jack cheese

---

COOK'S TIP ON FRESH CORN When cutting corn from the cob, place one end of the corn cob in the hole in the center of a tube pan or Bundt pan. As you cut downward, the corn kernels will fall into the pan.

PER SERVING

calories 224	cholesterol 2 mg	protein 7 g	dietary exchanges
total fat 5.5 g	sodium 37 mg	calcium 63 mg	2 starch
saturated 1.0 g	carbohydrates 41 g	potassium 430 mg	2 vegetable
trans 0.0 g	fiber 7 g		½ fat
polyunsaturated 1.0 g	sugars 5 g		
monounsaturated 3.0 g			

VEGETARIAN CASSOULET

Cassoulet is a stew typically made with beans and several kinds of meat, including sausage. In this version, however, extra vegetables stand in for the meat. The thick, herb-infused broth adds flavor, and fresh, crisp bread crumbs provide a little crunch in every bite.

SERVES 4 | 1½ cups per serving

In a large, deep skillet, heat 2 teaspoons oil over medium-high heat, swirling to coat the bottom. Cook the carrots, celery, and onion for 6 minutes, or until soft, stirring frequently.

Add the garlic. Cook for 1 minute, stirring constantly. Set aside.

Measure 1 cup beans into a medium bowl. Using a potato masher, mash until chunky. Stir the mashed beans, remaining whole beans, tomatoes with liquid, broth, thyme, pepper, and salt into the carrot mixture. Bring to a boil, still over medium-high heat. Reduce the heat and simmer, covered, for 20 minutes, or until the cassoulet is thickened.

Meanwhile, preheat the oven to 350°F.

In a small bowl, stir together the bread crumbs and remaining 2 teaspoons oil until the crumbs are moist. Spread in a small metal baking pan.

2 teaspoons olive oil and 2 teaspoons olive oil, divided use

2 large carrots, chopped

2 medium ribs of celery, chopped

1 large onion, chopped

2 medium garlic cloves, minced

2 15.5-ounce cans no-salt-added cannellini beans, rinsed and drained, divided use

1 14.5-ounce can no-salt-added diced tomatoes, undrained

1 cup Vegetable Broth (page 53) or commercial low-sodium vegetable broth

¾ teaspoon dried thyme, crumbled

¼ teaspoon pepper

¼ teaspoon salt

(continued)

Bake the bread-crumb mixture for 8 to 10 minutes, or until crisp, stirring once halfway through.

Remove the cassoulet from the heat. Stir in the parsley and lemon juice.

Just before serving, sprinkle with the bread-crumb mixture.

¾ cup fresh whole-wheat bread crumbs (from lowest-sodium-available bread)

2 tablespoons snipped fresh parsley

1 tablespoon fresh lemon juice

PER SERVING

calories 304
total fat 6.5 g
  saturated 0.5 g
  trans 0.0 g
  polyunsaturated 1.0 g
  monounsaturated 4.0 g

cholesterol 0 mg
sodium 324 mg
carbohydrates 48 g
  fiber 13 g
  sugars 11 g

protein 14 g
calcium 136 mg
potassium 962 mg

dietary exchanges
  2 starch
  3 vegetable
  ½ very lean meat
  1 fat

BRAISED LENTIL AND VEGETABLE MEDLEY

A blend of lentils, brown rice, winter squash, and aromatic vegetables, this dish is easy to prepare on the stovetop or in a slow cooker.

SERVES 4 | 1½ cups per serving

Using a vegetable peeler, peel the squash. Cut in half lengthwise with a large, sharp knife, discarding the seeds and strings. (Be careful; the squash is very hard and can slip.) Cut crosswise into ½-inch slices. Set aside.

In a large saucepan, heat the oil over medium heat, swirling to coat the bottom. Cook the mushrooms, bell pepper, onion, and garlic for 3 to 4 minutes, or until the bell pepper is tender-crisp and the onion is soft, stirring occasionally.

Stir in the squash. Cook for 2 to 3 minutes, or until the squash is slightly golden brown on the edges.

Stir in the broth, oregano, and pepper. Increase the heat to medium high and bring to a simmer, stirring occasionally.

Stir in the lentils. Reduce the heat and simmer, covered, for 30 to 35 minutes, or until the lentils and vegetables are tender, stirring occasionally.

Stir in the rice. Return to a simmer and simmer, covered, for 10 minutes, or until the rice is tender.

1 1¼-pound butternut squash

1 teaspoon olive oil

8 ounces medium brown (cremini) or button mushrooms, quartered

1 medium red bell pepper, thinly sliced

1 medium onion, thinly sliced

2 medium garlic cloves, minced

3½ cups Vegetable Broth (page 53) or commercial low-sodium vegetable broth

½ teaspoon dried oregano, crumbled

¼ teaspoon pepper

½ cup uncooked lentils, sorted for stones and shriveled lentils, rinsed, and drained

¾ cup uncooked instant brown rice

SLOW-COOKER METHOD

Put all the ingredients except the rice in a 3½- or 4-quart slow cooker. Cook on high for 2½ to 3½ hours or on low for 7½ to 9½ hours. Stir in the rice. Cook on either setting for 30 minutes, or until the lentils, vegetables, and rice are tender.

COOK'S TIP You can substitute 4 cups of your favorite winter squash, such as acorn, golden acorn, buttercup, or hubbard, for the butternut squash. If you prefer to use zucchini or yellow summer squash, you'll need about 1 pound.

PER SERVING

calories 246	**cholesterol** 0 mg	**protein** 12 g	**dietary exchanges**
total fat 2.5 g	**sodium** 36 mg	**calcium** 85 mg	3 starch
saturated 0.5 g	**carbohydrates** 48 g	**potassium** 938 mg	1 vegetable
trans 0.0 g	fiber 12 g		½ very lean meat
polyunsaturated 0.5 g	sugars 8 g		
monounsaturated 1.0 g			

SPINACH AND CHICKPEA KÖFTE with Yogurt Sauce

Köfte (*KAAF-tee*) are Turkish meatballs, usually made with lamb, herbs, and spices. This vegetarian version is sure to become a weeknight standby. Try it with steamed carrots and a romaine-based salad.

SERVES 4 | 2 köfte and 2 tablespoons sauce per serving

In a medium bowl, using a potato masher, coarsely mash the chickpeas. Stir in the remaining köfte ingredients except the oil. Divide the mixture into 8 balls. Lightly flatten each to about 2 inches in diameter.

In a large nonstick skillet, heat the oil over medium heat, swirling to coat the bottom. Cook the köfte for 2 to 3 minutes on each side, or until heated through and browned.

Meanwhile, in a small bowl, stir together the yogurt, parsley, and lemon juice. Spoon over the cooked köfte. Serve with the lemon wedges to squeeze on top.

KÖFTE

- 1 15.5-ounce can no-salt-added chickpeas, rinsed and drained
- 10 ounces frozen chopped spinach, thawed, well drained, and squeezed dry
- ¼ cup plain dry bread crumbs (lowest sodium available)
- 1 large egg white
- ½ teaspoon minced garlic
- ½ teaspoon ground cumin
- ⅛ teaspoon pepper
- 2 teaspoons olive oil

- ½ cup fat-free plain yogurt
- 1 tablespoon snipped fresh parsley
- 2 teaspoons fresh lemon juice
- 1 medium lemon, quartered

PER SERVING

calories 204	**cholesterol** 1 mg	**protein** 12 g	**dietary exchanges**
total fat 4.0 g	**sodium** 166 mg	**calcium** 214 mg	2 starch
saturated 0.5 g	**carbohydrates** 31 g	**potassium** 591 mg	1 lean meat
trans 0.0 g	fiber 7 g		
polyunsaturated 0.5 g	sugars 5 g		
monounsaturated 1.5 g			

STUFFED PEPPERS
with Brown Rice and Cannellini Beans

This vegetarian take on a classic uses brown rice instead of white, cannellini beans instead of ground beef, and an herby wine vinegar mixture instead of tomato sauce to fill roasted bell pepper halves.

SERVES 4 | 2 stuffed pepper halves per serving

In a medium saucepan, cook the rice using the package directions, omitting the salt and margarine.

Meanwhile, preheat the oven to 425°F. Lightly spray a 13 x 9 x 2-inch glass baking dish with cooking spray. Set aside.

Place the bell pepper halves with the cut side down in a single layer in another 13 x 9 x 2-inch glass baking dish (doesn't need to be sprayed).

Roast the peppers, covered, for about 20 minutes, or until tender-crisp. Using tongs, transfer the peppers with the cut side up to the sprayed baking dish. Set aside.

Reduce the oven temperature to 350°F.

Stir the remaining ingredients except the parsley into the cooked rice. Spoon about ¾ cup rice mixture into each pepper half.

Bake for 15 to 20 minutes, or until the mixture is heated through and the peppers are tender. Sprinkle with the parsley. Serve hot or at room temperature.

½ cup plus 2 tablespoons uncooked instant brown rice

Cooking spray

4 medium bell peppers, any color or combination, halved lengthwise

1 15.5-ounce can no-salt-added cannellini beans, rinsed and drained

2 medium ribs of celery, finely chopped

½ medium yellow onion, chopped

¼ cup red wine vinegar

1 tablespoon olive oil

1 teaspoon dried oregano, crumbled

1 teaspoon dried thyme, crumbled

1 teaspoon dried basil, crumbled

2 tablespoons snipped Italian (flat-leaf) parsley

PER SERVING

calories 217	**cholesterol** 0 mg	**protein** 8 g	**dietary exchanges**
total fat 5.0 g	**sodium** 60 mg	**calcium** 72 mg	2 starch
saturated 0.5 g	**carbohydrates** 35 g	**potassium** 582 mg	1 vegetable
trans 0.0 g	fiber 8 g		½ fat
polyunsaturated 0.5 g	sugars 7 g		
monounsaturated 2.5 g			

MOZZARELLA-QUINOA PATTIES with No-Cook Tomato Sauce

As these patties cook, the mozzarella cheese browns and creates a deliciously crisp crust. Prepare the sauce while the patties chill and let it stand at room temperature so the flavors blend.

SERVES 4 | 2 patties and ¼ cup sauce per serving

In a medium saucepan, stir together the water and quinoa. Bring to a boil over high heat. Reduce the heat and simmer, covered, for 12 to 15 minutes, or until the quinoa is tender and the liquid is absorbed.

Spread the quinoa in a thin layer on a large piece of wax paper. Let cool for about 10 minutes (you don't want it to be hot enough to cook the egg or melt the cheese). Transfer to a medium bowl.

Stir in the remaining ingredients for the patties.

Lightly coat a ¼ cup measuring cup with cooking spray. Spoon enough mixture into the measuring cup to lightly pack. Invert onto a small baking sheet. Repeat to make 7 more patties. Cover and refrigerate for 20 minutes.

Meanwhile, in a food processor or blender, process the sauce ingredients until coarsely chopped. Set aside.

PATTIES

1½ cups water

1 cup uncooked prerinsed quinoa

1 cup shredded or grated low-fat mozzarella cheese (about 4 ounces)

2 large egg whites

¼ cup plain dry bread crumbs (lowest sodium available)

⅛ teaspoon pepper

Cooking spray

2 teaspoons olive oil

SAUCE

1 large tomato (about 10 ounces), chopped

2 tablespoons chopped fresh basil

2 teaspoons fresh lemon juice

1 teaspoon olive oil

1 small garlic clove, minced

Pinch of pepper

In a large nonstick skillet, heat 2 teaspoons oil over medium heat, swirling to coat the bottom. Cook the chilled patties for 2 to 3 minutes on each side, or until heated through and browned.

Serve the sauce at room temperature with the patties.

PER SERVING

calories 286	**cholesterol** 10 mg	**protein** 16 g	**dietary exchanges**
total fat 9.0 g	**sodium** 284 mg	**calcium** 295 mg	2½ starch
saturated 2.0 g	**carbohydrates** 36 g	**potassium** 423 mg	1½ lean meat
trans 0.0 g	fiber 5 g		
polyunsaturated 2.0 g	sugars 2 g		
monounsaturated 4.0 g			

ASIAN VEGETABLE AND TOFU STIR-FRY

Colorful and quick, this stir-fry is tossed in hoisin sauce and toasted sesame oil, then served over brown rice and garnished with chopped nuts.

SERVES 4 | 1 cup vegetable and tofu mixture and ½ cup rice per serving

Put the cornstarch in a small bowl. Add the broth, hoisin sauce, soy sauce, and sesame oil, whisking until the cornstarch is dissolved. Set aside.

Prepare the rice using the package directions, omitting the salt and margarine.

Meanwhile, in a large saucepan, heat the canola oil over medium-high heat, swirling to coat the bottom. Cook the garlic for 15 to 20 seconds, or until soft, stirring occasionally and watching carefully so it doesn't burn.

Stir in the tofu. Cook for 3 to 4 minutes, or until light golden brown and heated through, stirring constantly.

Stir in the remaining ingredients except the peanuts. Cook for 2 to 3 minutes, or until the peas and bok choy are tender-crisp and the mixture is heated through, stirring constantly.

2 teaspoons cornstarch

¼ cup Vegetable Broth (page 53) or commercial low-sodium vegetable broth

2 tablespoons hoisin sauce

1 tablespoon soy sauce (lowest sodium available)

1 teaspoon toasted sesame oil

1 cup uncooked instant brown rice

1 teaspoon canola or corn oil

2 medium garlic cloves, minced

1 12.3-ounce package light extra-firm tofu, drained, patted dry, and cut into ½-inch cubes

4 ounces sugar snap peas, trimmed

4 medium stalks of bok choy (green and white parts), cut crosswise into ½-inch slices

(continued)

Make a well in the center of the tofu mixture. Pour in the reserved broth mixture. Bring to a simmer, still over medium-high heat, stirring constantly in the well only. Simmer for 2 to 3 minutes, or until the broth mixture is thickened, stirring constantly. Stir into the tofu mixture. Spoon over the rice. Sprinkle with the peanuts.

½ cup canned baby corn, drained

¼ cup canned sliced water chestnuts, drained

2 tablespoons chopped unsalted peanuts, other unsalted nuts, or sesame seeds

PER SERVING

calories 226	**cholesterol** 0 mg	**protein** 11 g	**dietary exchanges**
total fat 6.0 g	**sodium** 294 mg	**calcium** 82 mg	2 starch
saturated 0.5 g	**carbohydrates** 33 g	**potassium** 255 mg	1 lean meat
trans 0.0 g	fiber 3 g		
polyunsaturated 2.0 g	sugars 5 g		
monounsaturated 2.5 g			

CARROT, EDAMAME, AND BROWN RICE SKILLET

This recipe offers powerful nutrition, plus a pleasing mix of colors, shapes, and textures.

SERVES 4 | 1½ cups per serving

Prepare the rice using the package directions, omitting the salt and margarine.

In a medium nonstick skillet, heat the oil over medium-high heat, swirling to coat the bottom. Cook the onion and garlic for about 3 minutes, or until the onion is soft, stirring frequently.

Stir in the carrots, edamame, and bell pepper. Cook for 3 to 4 minutes, or until they are just tender, stirring frequently.

Stir in the rice, lemon juice, and thyme.

½ cup uncooked instant brown rice

2 teaspoons olive oil

½ cup chopped onion

1 medium garlic clove, minced

2 cups shredded carrots (4 to 5 medium)

¾ cup frozen shelled edamame (green soybeans)

1 medium red bell pepper, diced

3 tablespoons fresh lemon juice

1½ teaspoons finely snipped fresh thyme or ½ teaspoon dried, crumbled

PER SERVING

calories 144	**cholesterol** 0 mg	**protein** 6 g	**dietary exchanges**
total fat 4.0 g	**sodium** 45 mg	**calcium** 44 mg	1 starch
saturated 0.5 g	**carbohydrates** 21 g	**potassium** 403 mg	2 vegetable
trans 0.0 g	fiber 5 g		½ fat
polyunsaturated 0.5 g	sugars 6 g		
monounsaturated 2.0 g			

CRUSTLESS GARDEN QUICHE

For a rainy-night supper, serve this "sunshine on a plate."

SERVES 6 | 1 wedge per serving

Preheat the oven to 350°F. Lightly spray a 9-inch glass deep pie pan with cooking spray. Set aside.

In a large nonstick skillet, heat the oil over medium-high heat. Cook the mushrooms for 6 minutes, or until they begin to brown slightly, stirring frequently.

Stir in the bell pepper. Cook for 2 minutes, stirring frequently.

Meanwhile, in a medium bowl, whisk together the egg substitute, ¼ cup Cheddar, the milk, mustard, Worcestershire sauce, and cayenne. Set aside.

Spread the mushroom mixture in the pie pan. Top with the broccoli and cauliflower, parsley, and ¼ cup Cheddar. Pour the egg substitute mixture over all.

Bake for 30 minutes (the quiche won't be quite set). Sprinkle with the remaining ½ cup Cheddar. Bake for 5 minutes. Let stand for 5 minutes. Cut into 6 wedges.

Cooking spray

- 1 teaspoon canola or corn oil
- 8 ounces button mushrooms, sliced
- 1 medium red bell pepper, thinly sliced
- 1½ cups egg substitute
- ¼ cup shredded low-fat sharp Cheddar cheese, ¼ cup shredded low-fat sharp Cheddar cheese, and ½ cup shredded low-fat sharp Cheddar cheese, divided use
- ¼ cup fat-free evaporated milk
- 1 tablespoon Dijon mustard (lowest sodium available)
- ½ teaspoon Worcestershire sauce (lowest sodium available)
- ¼ teaspoon cayenne
- 10 ounces frozen broccoli and cauliflower, thawed and patted dry, large pieces halved
- ¼ cup snipped fresh parsley

PER SERVING

calories 109	**cholesterol** 4 mg	**protein** 14 g	**dietary exchanges**
total fat 2.5 g	**sodium** 320 mg	**calcium** 156 mg	1 vegetable
saturated 1.0 g	**carbohydrates** 8 g	**potassium** 411 mg	2 lean meat
trans 0.0 g	fiber 2 g		
polyunsaturated 0.5 g	sugars 5 g		
monounsaturated 1.0 g			

DOUBLE-SWISS QUICHE

Swiss chard and a Swiss-like (Jarlsberg) cheese combine to make a yummy crustless quiche. While it bakes, toss a salad to complete the meal.

SERVES 4 | 1 wedge per serving

Preheat the oven to 350°F. Lightly spray a 9-inch deep pie pan with cooking spray. Set aside.

In a large nonstick skillet, heat the oil over medium-high heat, swirling to coat the bottom. Cook the onion for 3 minutes, or until soft, stirring frequently.

Stir in the chard and garlic. Cook for 3 minutes, or until tender, stirring frequently. Stir in the sun-dried tomatoes. Remove from the heat and set aside.

In a large bowl, stir together the Swiss and Parmesan cheeses and the flour.

In a medium bowl, whisk together the remaining ingredients. Gradually add to the cheese mixture, stirring to combine. Stir in the chard mixture. Pour into the pie pan.

Bake for 55 minutes to 1 hour 5 minutes, or until a knife inserted in the center of the quiche comes out clean.

Cooking spray
- 1 teaspoon olive oil
- ¾ cup chopped onion (sweet, such as Vidalia, Maui, or Oso Sweet, preferred)
- 4 cups packed coarsely chopped green or red Swiss chard, thick stems discarded before measuring (about 3 large leaves or 6 to 8 ounces)
- 3 medium garlic cloves, minced
- 4 dry-packed sun-dried tomato halves, coarsely chopped
- 3 ¾-ounce slices (2¼ ounces total) low-fat Jarlsberg cheese, cut into 1-inch strips
- 3 tablespoons shredded or grated Parmesan cheese
- 3 tablespoons all-purpose flour
- 1 large egg
- ¾ cup egg substitute
- 1 cup fat-free milk
- ¼ cup fat-free half-and-half
- ⅛ teaspoon cayenne

COOK'S TIP ON SUN-DRIED TOMATOES Sun-dried tomatoes originated in Italy so people would be able to enjoy tomatoes during the winter. Ripe tomatoes are dried to remove most of their water content, deeply concentrating the flavor. It takes about 20 pounds of fresh tomatoes to yield just 1 pound of sun-dried tomatoes. Like fresh tomatoes, the sun-dried variety is a good source of vitamins. Use kitchen scissors to easily cut the tomatoes into small pieces.

PER SERVING

calories 188	**cholesterol** 65 mg	**protein** 18 g	**dietary exchanges**
total fat 5.5 g	**sodium** 364 mg	**calcium** 308 mg	½ starch
saturated 2.5 g	**carbohydrates** 17 g	**potassium** 522 mg	1 vegetable
trans 0.0 g	fiber 2 g		2 lean meat
polyunsaturated 0.5 g	sugars 7 g		
monounsaturated 2.0 g			

ZUCCHINI FRITTATA

Bursting with Italian flavor, this frittata is equally at home at brunch or dinner.

SERVES 4 | 1 wedge per serving

Preheat the oven to 350°F with the top rack about 4 inches from the heat.

In a large broilerproof nonstick skillet, heat the oil over medium heat, swirling to coat the bottom. Cook the zucchini for about 6 minutes, or until soft, stirring occasionally.

Stir in the green onions. Cook for 1 minute.

Stir in the tomatoes, garlic, Italian seasoning, and pepper. Cook for 5 minutes, or until the mixture has slightly thickened, stirring frequently.

Stir in the egg whites. Sprinkle with the mozzarella.

Bake for 12 minutes, or until a toothpick inserted in the center comes out clean. Leaving the pan in the oven, change the setting to broil. Broil for 3 to 4 minutes, or until golden brown. Sprinkle with the Parmesan. Cut into 4 wedges.

1 teaspoon canola or corn oil

1 medium zucchini, diced

3 medium green onions, sliced

1 14.5-ounce can no-salt-added tomatoes, drained

2 medium garlic cloves, minced

½ teaspoon dried Italian seasoning, crumbled

¼ teaspoon pepper

6 large egg whites or ¾ cup egg substitute, whites whisked to combine

½ cup shredded low-fat mozzarella cheese (about 2 ounces)

1 tablespoon shredded or grated Parmesan cheese

PER SERVING

calories 115	**cholesterol** 6 mg	**protein** 11 g	**dietary exchanges**
total fat 4.0 g	**sodium** 223 mg	**calcium** 186 mg	2 vegetable
saturated 1.0 g	**carbohydrates** 9 g	**potassium** 521 mg	1 lean meat
trans 0.0 g	fiber 3 g		
polyunsaturated 1.0 g	sugars 5 g		
monounsaturated 2.0 g			

CHEESE-TOPPED STUFFED EGGPLANT

Mild yet rich tasting, this easy-to-make dish gets a lot of Mediterranean flavor from the Greek seasoning blend and mozzarella and Parmesan cheeses.

SERVES 4 | 1 eggplant half and 1 cup filling per serving

Cooking spray

- 2 medium eggplants (about 1 pound each), trimmed and halved lengthwise
- 1 medium green bell pepper, finely chopped
- 1 large onion, finely chopped
- ½ cup water
- 1 tablespoon dried Greek seasoning
- 8 fat-free, low-sodium saltine crackers, crushed
- 1 8-ounce can no-salt-added tomato sauce
- ¼ cup snipped fresh parsley
- ⅛ teaspoon crushed red pepper flakes
- 1 cup shredded low-fat mozzarella cheese
- 1 tablespoon plus 1 teaspoon shredded or grated Parmesan cheese

Preheat the oven to 350°F. Lightly spray a Dutch oven and 13 x 9 x 2-inch baking pan with cooking spray. Set aside.

Leaving a ¼-inch rim, scoop out the eggplant pulp and transfer to a cutting board. Chop the eggplant pulp. Set it and the shells aside.

In the Dutch oven, cook the bell pepper and onion over medium-high heat for 4 minutes, or until the onion is soft, stirring frequently.

Stir in the chopped eggplant, water, and Greek seasoning. Reduce the heat to medium. Cook, covered, for 4 to 5 minutes, or until the eggplant is tender.

Stir in the cracker crumbs, tomato sauce, parsley, and red pepper flakes. Spoon into the eggplant shells. Place the shells in the baking pan. Sprinkle with the mozzarella.

Bake for 20 minutes, or until the mozzarella has melted and the shells are tender when pierced with a fork. Remove from the oven. Sprinkle with the Parmesan.

PER SERVING

calories 191	**cholesterol** 11 mg	**protein** 12 g	**dietary exchanges**
total fat 3.5 g	**sodium** 341 mg	**calcium** 323 mg	½ starch
saturated 1.5 g	**carbohydrates** 30 g	**potassium** 924 mg	5 vegetable
trans 0.0 g	fiber 11 g		1 lean meat
polyunsaturated 0.5 g	sugars 13 g		
monounsaturated 1.0 g			

RATATOUILLE-POLENTA CASSEROLE

Creamy, cheesy polenta tops a chunky mixture of vegetables in this hearty casserole.

SERVES 4 | 1½ cups per serving

Preheat the oven to 375°F. Lightly spray an 8-inch square glass baking dish with cooking spray.

In a large nonstick skillet, heat the oil over medium-high heat, swirling to coat the bottom. Cook the eggplant, onion, bell pepper, and garlic, covered, for 6 to 8 minutes, or until the eggplant is lightly browned and all the vegetables are softened, stirring occasionally.

Stir in the remaining filling ingredients. Cook, covered, for 5 minutes, or until the vegetables are tender, stirring frequently. Spoon into the baking dish.

Meanwhile, in a medium saucepan, bring the broth to a boil over medium-high heat. Using a long-handled whisk, carefully stir the broth to create a swirl. Slowly pour the cornmeal in a steady stream into the swirl, whisking constantly. Holding the pan steady, continue whisking for 1 to 2 minutes, or until the polenta is very thick. Remove from the heat.

Cooking spray

FILLING

2 teaspoons olive oil

1¼ pounds eggplant (about 1 medium), peeled and cut into ¾-inch cubes (about 6 cups)

1 medium onion, chopped

1 large red bell pepper, chopped

2 medium garlic cloves, minced

1 14.5-ounce can no-salt-added diced tomatoes, undrained

½ teaspoon dried basil, crumbled

½ teaspoon dried oregano, crumbled

⅛ teaspoon salt

⅛ teaspoon pepper

(continued)

Stir ½ cup Parmesan and the pepper into the polenta. Spread the polenta over the filling. Sprinkle with the remaining 2 tablespoons Parmesan.

Bake for 15 minutes, or until bubbling. Let the casserole stand for 5 minutes before serving.

POLENTA

2 cups Vegetable Broth (page 53) or commercial low-sodium vegetable broth

½ cup yellow cornmeal

½ cup shredded or grated Parmesan cheese and 2 tablespoons shredded or grated Parmesan cheese, divided use

⅛ teaspoon pepper

PER SERVING

calories 216	**cholesterol** 9 mg	**protein** 9 g	**dietary exchanges**
total fat 6.5 g	**sodium** 314 mg	**calcium** 208 mg	1 starch
saturated 2.5 g	**carbohydrates** 33 g	**potassium** 703 mg	3 vegetable
trans 0.0 g	fiber 7 g		½ very lean meat
polyunsaturated 0.5 g	sugars 10 g		1 fat
monounsaturated 3.0 g			

POTATO SKIN NACHOS

Using potatoes instead of tortilla chips as the base for beans, salsa, and other traditional nacho toppings helps you control your sodium intake. The potatoes are a good source of potassium, an important nutrient in helping lower blood pressure.

SERVES 4 | 4 nachos per serving

Preheat the oven to 375°F.

Put the potatoes on a nonstick baking sheet. Lightly spray the potatoes with olive oil spray. Sprinkle the potatoes with 1 teaspoon Chili Powder.

Bake for 30 minutes, or until the potatoes are tender when pierced with a fork.

Meanwhile, for the bean spread, in a medium skillet, heat the oil over medium-high heat, swirling to coat the bottom. Cook the onion and garlic for 3 minutes, or until the onion is soft, stirring frequently.

Stir in the remaining bean spread ingredients. Reduce the heat to medium. Cook the mixture for 1 minute, or until heated through, stirring occasionally. Spread on a large plate. Let cool for 5 to 10 minutes.

Meanwhile, in a medium bowl, stir together the salsa ingredients. Set aside.

POTATOES

4 4-ounce red potatoes, each cut into 4 wedges, or 1 pound whole fingerling potatoes

Olive oil spray

1 teaspoon Chili Powder (page 277) or no-salt-added chili powder

BEAN SPREAD

1 teaspoon olive oil

1 small onion, chopped

2 medium garlic cloves, minced

1 cup canned no-salt-added fat-free refried beans or 1 cup pureed canned no-salt-added pinto beans, rinsed and drained before pureeing

1 teaspoon Chili Powder (page 277) or no-salt-added chili powder

1 teaspoon very low sodium beef bouillon granules

⅛ teaspoon pepper

(continued)

Arrange the potatoes on a serving plate. Spread the bean spread over the potatoes. Spoon the salsa over the bean spread. Sprinkle with the Cheddar and olives. Top with the sour cream.

SALSA

2 medium Italian plum (Roma) tomatoes, chopped

½ medium bell pepper, any color, chopped

¼ cup chopped red onion

1 tablespoon snipped fresh cilantro or parsley

1 tablespoon chopped fresh jalapeño (optional)

TOPPING

½ cup fat-free shredded Cheddar cheese

2 tablespoons sliced black olives, drained

2 tablespoons fat-free sour cream

PER SERVING

calories 234
total fat 3.0 g
  saturated 0.5 g
  trans 0.0 g
  polyunsaturated 1.0 g
  monounsaturated 1.5 g

cholesterol 4 mg
sodium 191 mg
carbohydrates 41 g
  fiber 8 g
  sugars 6 g

protein 12 g
calcium 201 mg
potassium 1089 mg

dietary exchanges
2½ starch
1 vegetable
1 very lean meat

VEGETARIAN CHILI

When it's time to put logs in the fireplace, it's also time to fire up a big pot of this chili, flavored with lots of cumin and brightened with lemon juice.

SERVES 7 | 1½ cups per serving

Lightly spray a large saucepan with cooking spray. Put the oil in the pan, swirling to coat the bottom. Cook the onions, bell peppers, and garlic over medium-high heat for 8 to 10 minutes, or until the bell peppers are soft, stirring frequently. Reduce the heat if necessary to prevent burning.

Stir in the remaining ingredients except the beans. Reduce the heat and simmer, covered, for 45 minutes to 1 hour, or until the bulgur is done.

Stir in the beans. Simmer, uncovered, for 10 minutes.

Cooking spray
- 2 teaspoons canola or corn oil
- 2 large onions, chopped
- 2 medium green bell peppers, chopped
- 2 medium garlic cloves, minced
- 2 cups water
- 1 cup uncooked bulgur
- 1 cup no-salt-added canned diced tomatoes, undrained
- 2 tablespoons ground cumin
- 1½ tablespoons Chili Powder (page 277) or no-salt-added chili powder, or to taste
- 1 tablespoon fresh lemon juice
- ½ teaspoon pepper
- ¼ teaspoon cayenne
- 2 15.5-ounce cans no-salt-added kidney beans, rinsed and drained

PER SERVING

calories 237
total fat 2.5 g
  saturated 0.0 g
  trans 0.0 g
  polyunsaturated 0.5 g
  monounsaturated 1.0 g

cholesterol 0 mg
sodium 21 mg
carbohydrates 46 g
  fiber 11 g
  sugars 8 g

protein 12 g
calcium 121 mg
potassium 813 mg

dietary exchanges
2½ starch
2 vegetable
½ very lean meat

VEGETABLES & SIDE DISHES

TANGY ROASTED ASPARAGUS

Just a bit of Worcestershire is all it takes to give zing to this side dish.

SERVES 4 | 5 spears per serving

Preheat the oven to 425°F.

Line a baking sheet with aluminum foil. Lightly spray the foil with cooking spray. Arrange the asparagus in a single layer on the foil. Lightly spray the asparagus with cooking spray.

Roast for 10 minutes, or until just tender and beginning to brown lightly on the tips.

In a small saucepan, stir together the remaining ingredients. Cook over medium heat for 1 minute, or just until the margarine melts. Stir. Drizzle over the asparagus. Gently roll the asparagus to coat.

Cooking spray

1 pound asparagus spears (about 20), trimmed and patted dry

1 tablespoon light tub margarine

1 teaspoon fresh lemon juice

½ teaspoon Worcestershire sauce (lowest sodium available)

⅛ teaspoon salt

COOK'S TIP Be sure to pat the asparagus spears dry before placing them on the baking sheet. Otherwise they won't roast, and the taste of the dish will be altered.

PER SERVING

calories 35	**cholesterol** 0 mg	**protein** 2 g	**dietary exchanges**
total fat 1.0 g	**sodium** 96 mg	**calcium** 25 mg	1 vegetable
saturated 0.0 g	**carbohydrates** 5 g	**potassium** 284 mg	
trans 0.0 g	fiber 2 g		
polyunsaturated 0.5 g	sugars 3 g		
monounsaturated 0.5 g			

BARLEY AND CHARD PILAF

Oregano, shallots, and lemon juice enhance the vegetables in this barley-based dish. You can replace the chard with other greens, such as spinach, turnip greens, or collard greens, if you prefer, adjusting the cooking time as needed.

SERVES 4 | ½ cup per serving

In a medium saucepan, bring 1 cup water to a boil over high heat. Stir in the barley, oregano, and pepper. Reduce the heat and simmer, covered, for 10 to 12 minutes, or until the barley is tender and the water is absorbed.

In another medium saucepan, bring the remaining ¼ cup water to a boil over high heat. Stir in the chard. Reduce the heat and simmer, covered, for 5 to 8 minutes, or until the chard is tender. Drain well in a colander. Set aside.

Pour the oil into the pan the chard was in. Heat over medium-high heat, swirling to coat the bottom. Cook the shallots and bell pepper for 4 minutes, or until tender, stirring frequently.

Stir in the tomatoes, lemon juice, chard, and barley. Cook, uncovered, for 1 minute, or until the tomatoes are hot, stirring frequently.

- 1 cup water and ¼ cup water, divided use
- ½ cup uncooked quick-cooking barley
- ½ teaspoon dried oregano, crumbled, or 2 teaspoons snipped fresh
- ¼ teaspoon pepper
- 4 ounces red or green Swiss chard, tough stems discarded and leaves coarsely chopped (about 2 cups)
- 1 teaspoon olive oil
- 2 medium shallots, finely chopped
- ¼ cup finely chopped red bell pepper
- ⅓ cup chopped seeded tomatoes, drained
- 1 tablespoon fresh lemon juice

PER SERVING

calories 91	**cholesterol** 0 mg	**protein** 3 g	**dietary exchanges**
total fat 1.5 g	**sodium** 66 mg	**calcium** 30 mg	1 starch
saturated 0.5 g	**carbohydrates** 18 g	**potassium** 246 mg	
trans 0.0 g	fiber 3 g		
polyunsaturated 0.5 g	sugars 2 g		
monounsaturated 1.0 g			

BALSAMIC BEETS AND WALNUTS

Garnet-colored beets topped with a reduction of balsamic vinegar and brown sugar, then sprinkled with cinnamon-sugar walnuts, are a great complement to dishes such as Tarragon Turkey Medallions (page 161) or a simple roasted pork tenderloin.

SERVES 6 | ½ cup per serving

If using fresh beets, simmer in 2 quarts boiling water, covered, for 40 to 50 minutes, or until tender. Drain the beets and let cool for about 5 minutes, or until cool enough to handle. Slip the skins off. Cut the beets crosswise into ¼-inch slices.

If using canned beets, stir them and the water together in a medium microwaveable bowl. Microwave, covered, on 100 percent power (high) for 2 to 3 minutes, or until the beets are heated through. Drain.

Pour the beets into a serving bowl. Cover to keep warm. Set aside.

Meanwhile, in a small saucepan, stir together the vinegar and 1 tablespoon brown sugar. Bring to a simmer over medium-high heat, stirring constantly until the sugar is dissolved. Simmer for 6 to 8 minutes, or until the mixture is reduced by half, to about ¼ cup, without stirring. Remove from the heat. Set aside.

2 pounds fresh beets, all but 1 to 2 inches of stems discarded, or 2 15-ounce cans no-salt-added sliced beets, drained

2 tablespoons water (for canned beets)

½ cup balsamic vinegar

1 tablespoon light brown sugar and 1 teaspoon light brown sugar, divided use

Cooking spray

¼ cup walnut halves

¼ teaspoon ground cinnamon

⅛ teaspoon ground nutmeg

Lightly spray a small skillet with cooking spray. Stir together the walnuts, cinnamon, and nutmeg. Cook over medium-low heat for 2 to 3 minutes, or until the walnuts are lightly toasted, stirring occasionally. Stir in the remaining 1 teaspoon brown sugar. Cook for 1 to 2 minutes, or until the mixture is heated through (the sugar will still be somewhat granulated).

Drizzle the vinegar mixture over the beets. Sprinkle with the walnut mixture.

PER SERVING

calories 101	**cholesterol** 0 mg	**protein** 2 g	**dietary exchanges**
total fat 3.0 g	**sodium** 85 mg	**calcium** 27 mg	2 vegetable
saturated 0.5 g	**carbohydrates** 18 g	**potassium** 366 mg	½ other carbohydrate
trans 0.0 g	fiber 3 g		½ fat
polyunsaturated 2.0 g	sugars 14 g		
monounsaturated 0.5 g			

GREEN BEANS AND CORN

This pairing of two all-time favorite vegetables is simple but colorful.

SERVES 4 | ½ cup per serving

In a medium saucepan, bring the water to a boil over high heat. Stir in the beans and corn. Reduce the heat and simmer, covered, for 5 to 8 minutes, or until the beans are just tender. Drain well in a colander. Set aside.

In the same pan, melt the margarine over medium-high heat, swirling to coat the bottom. Cook the onion for 3 minutes, or until soft, stirring frequently.

Return the green beans and corn to the pan. Stir in the basil, lemon juice, and pepper.

½ cup water

1 cup sliced fresh green beans or frozen French-style green beans, trimmed if fresh

1 cup fresh or frozen whole-kernel corn

1 teaspoon light tub margarine

3 tablespoons chopped onion

½ teaspoon dried basil, crumbled

½ teaspoon fresh lemon juice

Dash of pepper

SUCCOTASH

Substitute fresh or frozen lima beans for the green beans. Increase the simmering time to 15 to 20 minutes. Substitute crumbled dried marjoram for the basil.

BAKED BEANS

No potluck meal or barbecue is complete without baked beans. These cook for a long time but need very little attention. The result is well worth the wait.

SERVES 6 | ½ cup per serving

In a Dutch oven, bring the water and beans to a boil over high heat. Boil for 2 minutes. Remove from the heat and let stand for 1 hour. Return to the heat and bring to a simmer over high heat. Reduce the heat and simmer, covered, for 1 hour, or until tender. Rinse and drain well in a colander.

Preheat the oven to 350°F. Lightly spray a 1½-quart casserole dish with cooking spray. Set aside.

In a small nonstick skillet, cook the pork chop over medium-high heat for 2 to 3 minutes on each side, or until browned. Cut into small cubes.

Pour the beans into the casserole dish. Stir in the pork, Chili Sauce, 1 cup water, the onion, molasses, brown sugar, mustard, and garlic powder.

Bake, covered, for 4 hours, or until the pork is tender. If the beans begin to dry out, stir in more water, about ¼ cup at a time.

4 cups water

8 ounces dried navy beans (about 1 cup), sorted for stones and shriveled beans, rinsed, and drained

Cooking spray

1 4-ounce loin-end pork chop, all visible fat discarded

1 cup Chili Sauce (page 276), or 1 cup no-salt-added ketchup plus dash of red hot-pepper sauce

1 cup water (plus more as needed)

1 medium onion, chopped

2 tablespoons dark or light molasses

1 tablespoon light brown sugar

1½ teaspoons dry mustard

¼ teaspoon garlic powder

PER SERVING

calories 236	**cholesterol** 10 mg	**protein** 11 g	**dietary exchanges**
total fat 3.0 g	**sodium** 32 mg	**calcium** 106 mg	2 starch
saturated 0.5 g	**carbohydrates** 43 g	**potassium** 749 mg	1 other carbohydrate
trans 0.0 g	fiber 11 g		1 very lean meat
polyunsaturated 0.5 g	sugars 18 g		
monounsaturated 1.0 g			

ROASTED BROCCOLI
with Onions

Roasting brings out the best flavor in both the broccoli florets and the onion slices in this side dish.

SERVES 4 | heaping ½ cup per serving

Preheat the oven to 400°F. Lightly spray a large shallow metal baking pan with cooking spray.

Put the onion in the baking pan. Drizzle with 1 teaspoon oil. Toss to coat. Spread the onion in a single layer.

Roast for 10 minutes. Remove from the oven. Stir the onion.

Meanwhile, in a medium bowl, combine the broccoli and remaining 1 teaspoon oil, tossing to coat. Stir into the roasted onion.

Roast for 10 minutes. Stir. Roast for 5 minutes, or until the onion and broccoli are tender and browned. Transfer to a medium bowl.

Add the lemon juice and salt, tossing to coat.

Cooking spray
- 1 **large onion (about 8 ounces), sliced lengthwise**
- 1 **teaspoon olive oil and 1 teaspoon olive oil, divided use**
- 3 **cups broccoli florets (in 2-inch pieces)**
- 1 **teaspoon fresh lemon juice**
- ⅛ **teaspoon salt**

PER SERVING

calories 58	**cholesterol** 0 mg	**protein** 2 g	**dietary exchanges**
total fat 2.5 g	**sodium** 97 mg	**calcium** 41 mg	2 vegetable
saturated 0.5 g	**carbohydrates** 8 g	**potassium** 272 mg	½ fat
trans 0.0 g	fiber 2 g		
polyunsaturated 0.5 g	sugars 3 g		
monounsaturated 1.5 g			

BRUSSELS SPROUTS
with Caramelized Onions and Fennel

The flavors of the fennel and caramelized onion make this unusual dish a standout.

SERVES 4 | ½ cup per serving

In a medium skillet, melt the margarine over medium-high heat, swirling to coat the bottom. Cook the onion for 2 minutes, stirring frequently. Reduce the heat to low. Cook, covered, for 5 minutes, or until the onion is soft.

Stir in the sugar and salt. Increase the heat to medium high. Stir in the fennel. Cook, uncovered, for 10 minutes, stirring occasionally. Cook for 5 to 10 minutes, or until the onion and fennel are golden brown and the fennel is tender, stirring frequently to prevent sticking.

Meanwhile, put the brussels sprouts in a medium saucepan. Pour in water to cover. Bring to a boil over medium-high heat. Boil for 6 to 8 minutes, or until tender. Drain in a colander. Transfer to a medium bowl. Set aside.

Stir the onion mixture into the brussels sprouts. Sprinkle with the walnuts.

- 2 teaspoons light tub margarine
- 1 large yellow onion, halved and thinly sliced into half-rings
- 1 teaspoon sugar
- ⅛ teaspoon salt
- 1 medium fennel bulb, trimmed, cut into matchstick-size pieces (about 1½ cups)
- 8 ounces small or medium brussels sprouts, whole if small or halved if medium, trimmed
- 2 tablespoons chopped walnuts, dry-roasted

PER SERVING

calories 92	**cholesterol** 0 mg	**protein** 4 g	**dietary exchanges**
total fat 3.5 g	**sodium** 134 mg	**calcium** 65 mg	3 vegetable
saturated 0.5 g	**carbohydrates** 14 g	**potassium** 534 mg	½ fat
trans 0.0 g	fiber 5 g		
polyunsaturated 2.0 g	sugars 4 g		
monounsaturated 1.0 g			

BULGUR PILAF
with Kale and Tomatoes

Enjoy a combination of nutritious vegetables and a whole grain all in one easy side dish. It goes equally well with Broiled Sirloin with Chile-Roasted Onions (page 176), Herb Chicken with Panko-Pecan Crust (page 148), or Wine-Poached Salmon (page 109).

SERVES 4 | ¾ cup per serving

In a large skillet, heat the oil over medium-high heat, swirling to coat the bottom. Cook the onion for 3 minutes, or until soft, stirring frequently.

Stir in the broth, kale, bulgur, garlic, pepper, and salt. Bring to a boil, still over medium-high heat. Reduce the heat and simmer, covered, for 12 minutes, or until the bulgur is tender and most of the liquid is absorbed, stirring occasionally.

Stir in the tomato. Cook for 1 minute, or until heated through. Remove from the heat. Stir in the lemon juice.

2 teaspoons olive oil

1 small onion, thinly sliced lengthwise

2 cups Chicken Broth (page 50) or commercial fat-free, low-sodium chicken broth

2 cups chopped kale

¾ cup uncooked bulgur

1 medium garlic clove, minced

¼ teaspoon pepper

⅛ teaspoon salt

1 medium Italian plum (Roma) tomato, chopped

2 tablespoons fresh lemon juice

COOK'S TIP Instead of the kale, you can use spinach in this recipe. Add the spinach with the tomato, stirring just until the spinach wilts.

PER SERVING

calories 149	cholesterol 0 mg	protein 6 g	dietary exchanges
total fat 3.0 g	sodium 124 mg	calcium 66 mg	1½ starch
saturated 0.5 g	carbohydrates 28 g	potassium 354 mg	1 vegetable
trans 0.0 g	fiber 6 g		½ fat
polyunsaturated 0.5 g	sugars 2 g		
monounsaturated 1.5 g			

CREAMY CARROTS
with Pecans

Be sure to use regular-size carrots, not baby carrots, for the proper sweetness and moisture in this delicate, lighter substitute for mashed sweet potatoes.

SERVES 4 | ½ cup per serving

In a large saucepan, steam the carrots for 15 minutes, or until very tender.

In a food processor or blender, process all the ingredients except the pecans until smooth, scraping the bottom and side occasionally. Transfer to a shallow dish. Sprinkle with the pecans.

- 1 pound carrots, cut crosswise into ½-inch slices
- ⅓ cup fat-free half-and-half
- 3 tablespoons firmly packed dark brown sugar
- 2 tablespoons light tub margarine
- ½ teaspoon vanilla, butter, and nut flavoring or vanilla extract
- 1 tablespoon finely chopped pecans, dry roasted (optional)

PER SERVING
WITH PECANS

calories 133
total fat 3.5 g
  saturated 0.0 g
  trans 0.0 g
  polyunsaturated 1.0 g
  monounsaturated 2.0 g

cholesterol 0 mg
sodium 146 mg
carbohydrates 24 g
  fiber 3 g
  sugars 17 g

protein 3 g
calcium 74 mg
potassium 388 mg

dietary exchanges
2 vegetable
1 other carbohydrate
1 fat

THYME-FLAVORED CAULIFLOWER

Here's the answer to what to do with cauliflower besides covering it with cheese sauce. Serve this alternative with Pork Chops with Herb Rub (page 196) and cinnamon applesauce.

SERVES 4 | ½ cup per serving

In a medium saucepan, bring a small amount of water (this is not the 2 tablespoons) to a boil over high heat. Boil fresh cauliflower, covered, for 10 to 12 minutes, or until just tender. If using frozen cauliflower, prepare using the package directions, omitting the salt. Drain well in a colander. Return to the pan.

Meanwhile, in a medium bowl, stir together 2 tablespoons water, the vinegar, garlic, thyme, and pepper. Set aside.

When the cauliflower is ready, stir in the vinegar mixture. Cook, covered, for 5 to 8 minutes, or until the cauliflower is tender. Serve sprinkled with the parsley.

1 medium cauliflower (about 1½ pounds), broken into small florets, or 10 ounces frozen cauliflower florets

2 tablespoons water

¾ to 1½ teaspoons cider vinegar

½ medium garlic clove, minced

¼ teaspoon dried thyme, crumbled

Dash of pepper

2 teaspoons finely snipped fresh parsley or 1 teaspoon dried, crumbled

PER SERVING

calories 37	**cholesterol** 0 mg	**protein** 3 g	**dietary exchanges**
total fat 0.0 g	**sodium** 44 mg	**calcium** 34 mg	2 vegetable
saturated 0.0 g	**carbohydrates** 8 g	**potassium** 442 mg	
trans 0.0 g	fiber 4 g		
polyunsaturated 0.0 g	sugars 4 g		
monounsaturated 0.0 g			

EGGPLANT MEXICANA

Want a tasty new way to get vegetables into your diet? Try this eggplant and tomato side dish, which gets a flavor burst from chili powder and fresh cilantro.

SERVES 8 | ½ cup per serving

In a large nonstick skillet, stir together all the ingredients except the cilantro. Bring to a simmer over medium heat. Reduce the heat and simmer, covered, for 15 to 20 minutes, or until the eggplant is tender. Serve sprinkled with the cilantro.

1 medium eggplant (about 1 pound), peeled and cubed

4 medium tomatoes, chopped, or 1 14.5-ounce can no-salt-added diced tomatoes, undrained

2 tablespoons chopped onion

1 medium garlic clove, minced

¼ to ½ teaspoon Chili Powder (page 277) or commercial no-salt-added chili powder

¼ teaspoon pepper

2 tablespoons snipped fresh cilantro or parsley

PER SERVING

calories 27	cholesterol 0 mg	protein 1 g	dietary exchanges
total fat 0.5 g	sodium 5 mg	calcium 14 mg	1 vegetable
saturated 0.0 g	carbohydrates 6 g	potassium 287 mg	
trans 0.0 g	fiber 3 g		
polyunsaturated 0.0 g	sugars 3 g		
monounsaturated 0.0 g			

GREENS with Tomatoes and Parmesan

The vibrant color contrast between the greens and the tomatoes adds eye appeal to this tasty dish.

SERVES 4 | heaping ½ cup per serving

Fill a Dutch oven half-full of water. Bring to a boil over high heat. Drop the greens into the water and cook for 5 to 8 minutes, or until tender. Drain well in a colander, being sure to drain off all the excess liquid.

In a large nonstick skillet, heat the oil over medium-high heat, swirling to coat the bottom. Stir in the greens, tomatoes, garlic, and Italian seasoning. Cook for 3 to 5 minutes, or until the tomatoes are heated through, stirring frequently. Sprinkle with the Parmesan.

1 large bunch (about 1 pound) collard greens or red or green Swiss chard, stems discarded, cut crosswise into large pieces

2 teaspoons olive oil

2 medium tomatoes, each cut into 8 wedges

2 medium garlic cloves, minced

½ teaspoon Italian seasoning, crumbled

2 to 3 tablespoons shredded or grated Parmesan cheese

COOK'S TIP After discarding the stems of the collard greens or Swiss chard, stack several leaves before cutting them. Repeat with the remaining leaves.

PER SERVING

calories 76	**cholesterol** 2 mg	**protein** 4 g	**dietary exchanges**
total fat 3.5 g	**sodium** 168 mg	**calcium** 171 mg	2 vegetable
saturated 1.0 g	**carbohydrates** 9 g	**potassium** 314 mg	1 fat
trans 0.0 g	fiber 5 g		
polyunsaturated 0.5 g	sugars 2 g		
monounsaturated 2.0 g			

ROASTED PLUMS
with Walnut Crunch

Is this recipe for a side dish or a dessert? It's your call—either way provides a serving of fruit for each diner. You might want to make a double batch of the walnut crunch and use the extra to top fat-free yogurt or hot cereal for breakfast.

SERVES 8 | ½ cup fruit and 1½ tablespoons crunch per serving

Preheat the oven to 400°F.

Put the plums with the skin side down in an 8-inch square glass baking dish. Cover a medium plate with cooking parchment. Set aside.

In a small bowl, stir together the orange juice, 2 tablespoons brown sugar, and ½ teaspoon cinnamon until the sugar is dissolved. Drizzle over the plums. Stir to coat.

Roast for 20 minutes, or until the plums are hot and just tender, stirring gently halfway through.

Meanwhile, for the crunch, melt the margarine in a small ovenproof skillet over medium heat. Stir in the remaining 2 tablespoons brown sugar. Cook for 2 minutes, or until the sugar is dissolved, stirring frequently.

Stir in the walnuts and remaining ½ teaspoon cinnamon. Add the oats, stirring to coat. Cook for 1 minute, stirring frequently.

PLUMS
- 2 pounds plums, any color or combination, quartered
- ⅓ cup fresh orange juice
- 2 tablespoons packed light brown sugar
- ½ teaspoon ground cinnamon

CRUNCH
- 2 teaspoons light tub margarine
- 2 tablespoons packed light brown sugar
- 2 tablespoons chopped walnuts, dry-roasted
- ½ teaspoon ground cinnamon
- ⅓ cup uncooked rolled oats

Bake the crunch for 5 minutes, or until the oats are toasted. Remove the skillet from the oven. Stir the crunch well. Pour onto the plate with the cooking parchment. Let stand for 8 to 10 minutes, or until cool.

Spoon the plums with juices into bowls. Top each serving with about 3 tablespoons of the crunch.

COOK'S TIP You can make the walnut crunch up to three days in advance. Prepare the crunch as directed and let it cool completely. Store it in an airtight container at room temperature.

PER SERVING

calories 109	**cholesterol** 0 mg	**protein** 2 g	**dietary exchanges**
total fat 2.0 g	**sodium** 10 mg	**calcium** 18 mg	1 fruit
saturated 0.0 g	**carbohydrates** 23 g	**potassium** 220 mg	½ other carbohydrate
trans 0.0 g	fiber 2 g		½ fat
polyunsaturated 1.0 g	sugars 18 g		
monounsaturated 0.5 g			

ROASTED RED PEPPERS AND PORTOBELLO MUSHROOMS

Since you serve this side dish at room temperature, it's perfect for a party or holiday buffet. It's also a terrific appetizer when served on crostini or low-sodium whole-grain crackers.

SERVES 12 | ½ cup per serving

Lightly spray the mushrooms with olive oil spray. Lightly spray a large indoor grill pan or grill rack with olive oil spray. Heat the pan for several minutes over medium-high heat or preheat the grill on medium high.

Grill the mushrooms for about 30 minutes, or until juicy. (The cooking time will vary depending on the size of the mushrooms. If you cook them too long, they will dry out.) Transfer to a cutting board. Slice to the desired thickness.

In a large bowl, stir together the mushrooms and roasted peppers.

In a small bowl, whisk together the vinegar and sugar until the sugar is dissolved. Pour over the mushroom mixture. Stir gently. Serve at room temperature.

4 medium portobello mushrooms, stems discarded

Olive oil spray

1½ cups roasted red bell peppers, sliced

¼ cup plain rice vinegar

2 teaspoons sugar, or to taste

PER SERVING

calories 12	**cholesterol** 0 mg	**protein** 1 g	**dietary exchanges** free
total fat 0.0 g	**sodium** 1 mg	**calcium** 3 mg	
saturated 0.0 g	**carbohydrates** 2 g	**potassium** 101 mg	
trans 0.0 g	fiber 0 g		
polyunsaturated 0.0 g	sugars 1 g		
monounsaturated 0.0 g			

SCALLOPED POTATOES

You'll attract an audience when you take these yummy potatoes out of the oven. The star of the meal, they go well with almost anything. Try them with grilled flank steak and zucchini.

SERVES 8 | ½ cup per serving

Preheat the oven to 350°F. Lightly spray a 1½-quart casserole dish with cooking spray. Set aside.

In a medium saucepan, whisk together the milk and flour. Whisk in the broth, pepper, onion powder, and garlic powder. Cook over medium-high heat for 5 to 6 minutes, or until thickened, whisking occasionally.

Whisk in the Parmesan. Remove from the heat.

In the casserole dish, stir together the potatoes and onion. Pour in the sauce, gently stirring to combine.

Bake, covered, for 30 minutes. Gently stir in the Cheddar. Sprinkle with the paprika. Bake, uncovered, for 30 to 40 minutes, or until the potatoes are tender and lightly browned.

Cooking spray
- 1 cup fat-free milk
- 3 tablespoons all-purpose flour
- 1 cup Chicken Broth (page 50) or commercial fat-free, low-sodium broth
- ¼ teaspoon pepper
- ¼ teaspoon onion powder
- ¼ teaspoon garlic powder
- 3 tablespoons shredded or grated Parmesan cheese
- 4 large potatoes, peeled and thinly sliced (about 4 cups)
- ½ cup chopped onion
- ½ cup low-fat shredded Cheddar cheese (about 2 ounces)
- ⅛ teaspoon paprika

PER SERVING

calories 176	**cholesterol** 3 mg	**protein** 7 g	**dietary exchanges**
total fat 1.0 g	**sodium** 99 mg	**calcium** 107 mg	2½ starch
saturated 0.5 g	**carbohydrates** 35 g	**potassium** 580 mg	½ very lean meat
trans 0.0 g	fiber 3 g		
polyunsaturated 0.0 g	sugars 3 g		
monounsaturated 0.5 g			

ZESTY OVEN-FRIED POTATOES

This is finger food at its finest! Invite some friends over for a meal of these oven-fries, stovetop pork chops, and Balsamic-Marinated Vegetables (page 78).

SERVES 6 | ½ cup per serving

Preheat the oven to 400°F. Lightly spray a large baking sheet with cooking spray.

Arrange the potato wedges in a single layer on the baking sheet.

In a small bowl, stir together the oil, Creole Seasoning, and pepper. Drizzle over the potatoes, stirring to coat.

Bake for 30 minutes, or until the potatoes are golden and tender.

Just before serving, sprinkle with the vinegar.

Cooking spray

1½ pounds medium red potatoes (4 to 5), each potato cut lengthwise into 6 wedges

1 tablespoon olive oil

½ to ¾ teaspoon Creole Seasoning (page 278) or salt-free spicy seasoning blend

½ teaspoon pepper

2 tablespoons malt vinegar

PER SERVING

calories 105	**cholesterol** 0 mg	**protein** 2 g	**dietary exchanges**
total fat 2.5 g	**sodium** 0 mg	**calcium** 17 mg	1½ starch
saturated 0.5 g	**carbohydrates** 20 g	**potassium** 483 mg	
trans 0.0 g	fiber 2 g		
polyunsaturated 0.0 g	sugars 1 g		
monounsaturated 1.5 g			

CITRUS AND MINT QUINOA
with Feta Crumbles

Quinoa, an excellent source of protein that counts toward your whole-grain goal, is the base for this citrusy side. Be sure to use fresh mint leaves— dried mint won't provide the flavor boost you want for this dish.

SERVES 4 | ½ cup per serving

In a small saucepan, stir together the orange juice, water, and quinoa. Bring to a boil over high heat. Reduce the heat and simmer, covered, for 12 to 15 minutes, or until the quinoa is tender and the liquid is absorbed. Remove from the heat. Fluff the quinoa with a fork. Let stand, covered, for 10 minutes.

Meanwhile, in a medium bowl, stir together the oil and lemon juice. Stir in the remaining ingredients except the feta. Set aside.

When the quinoa is ready, use a fork to lightly stir it into the oil mixture. Gently fold in the feta. Serve at room temperature.

½ cup fresh orange juice

½ cup water

½ cup uncooked prerinsed quinoa

1 teaspoon olive oil (extra virgin preferred)

2 tablespoons fresh lemon juice

1 tablespoon grated lemon zest

2 tablespoons golden raisins

1½ tablespoons finely chopped fresh mint

1 tablespoon snipped fresh Italian (flat-leaf) parsley

1 tablespoon sliced green onion

¼ cup crumbled low-fat feta cheese

PER SERVING

calories 139
total fat 3.5 g
  saturated 1.0 g
  trans 0.0 g
  polyunsaturated 1.0 g
  monounsaturated 1.5 g

cholesterol 3 mg
sodium 129 mg
carbohydrates 23 g
  fiber 2 g
  sugars 6 g

protein 5 g
calcium 74 mg
potassium 242 mg

dietary exchanges
1 starch
½ fruit
½ fat

RICE AND VEGETABLE PILAF

Full of mushrooms and carrots, this dish tastes great with Herbed Fillet of Sole (page 118).

SERVES 6 | ½ cup per serving

In a medium saucepan, heat the oil over medium-high heat, swirling to coat the bottom. Cook the mushrooms and carrots for 2 to 3 minutes, or until the mushrooms are soft, stirring occasionally.

Stir in the broth and pepper. Increase the heat to high and bring to a boil.

Stir in the rice. Reduce the heat and simmer, covered, for 20 minutes. Remove from the heat.

Stir in the parsley and green onions. Let stand for 5 minutes. Fluff with a fork before serving.

1 teaspoon olive oil

4 ounces button mushrooms, sliced

2 medium carrots, shredded

1 cup Chicken Broth (page 50) or commercial fat-free, low-sodium chicken broth

¼ teaspoon pepper

½ cup uncooked rice

½ cup snipped fresh parsley

2 medium green onions, sliced

PER SERVING

calories 78	**cholesterol** 0 mg	**protein** 2 g	**dietary exchanges**
total fat 1.0 g	**sodium** 26 mg	**calcium** 17 mg	1 starch
saturated 0.0 g	**carbohydrates** 16 g	**potassium** 206 mg	
trans 0.0 g	fiber 1 g		
polyunsaturated 0.0 g	sugars 2 g		
monounsaturated 0.5 g			

ASIAN FRIED RICE
with Peas

This dish is an excellent accompaniment to almost any Asian entrée, such as Chicken with Ginger and Snow Peas (page 157) or Pacific Rim Flank Steak (page 180). Add some chicken, shrimp, beef, or pork cooked without salt to transform this into a main dish.

SERVES 8 | ½ cup per serving

Prepare the rice using the package directions, omitting the salt and margarine. Spread on a baking sheet and refrigerate for at least 1 hour. For best results, transfer the cooked rice to an airtight container instead of to a baking sheet. Refrigerate for a day or so.

In a large nonstick skillet, heat the oil over medium-high heat, swirling to coat the bottom. Cook 4 or 5 green onions for 1 minute, or until fragrant, stirring occasionally.

Stir in the cilantro and rice. Cook for 2 minutes, or until heated, stirring constantly to separate the grains.

Stir in the vinegar, soy sauce, cumin, and sugar. Stir in the green peas. Cook for 2 to 3 minutes, or until the mixture is hot and the peas are heated through, stirring occasionally. Sprinkle with the remaining 2 green onions, then with the black sesame seeds.

- 1 cup uncooked brown rice or 4 cups well-chilled cooked brown rice
- 1 tablespoon canola or corn oil
- 4 or 5 medium green onions, thinly sliced, and 2 medium green onions, thinly sliced (optional), divided use
- 2 tablespoons snipped fresh cilantro
- 1½ tablespoons plain rice vinegar
- 1 tablespoon soy sauce (lowest sodium available)
- 1 teaspoon ground cumin
- ½ teaspoon sugar
- 1 cup frozen green peas
- 2 teaspoons black sesame seeds (optional)

PER SERVING

calories 146	**cholesterol** 0 mg	**protein** 4 g	**dietary exchanges**
total fat 3.0 g	**sodium** 75 mg	**calcium** 16 mg	2 starch
saturated 0.5 g	**carbohydrates** 26 g	**potassium** 118 mg	
trans 0.0 g	fiber 3 g		
polyunsaturated 1.0 g	sugars 2 g		
monounsaturated 1.5 g			

PARMESAN-LEMON SPINACH

A light cream sauce enhanced with Parmesan cheese coats fresh spinach in this side dish. Try it with pork chops, fish fillets, or turkey cutlets.

SERVES 4 | ½ cup per serving

In a medium bowl, whisk together the half-and-half, Parmesan, and flour until smooth. Set aside.

In a large nonstick skillet, heat the oil over medium heat, swirling to coat the bottom. Cook the shallots for 2 to 3 minutes, or until tender-crisp, stirring occasionally.

Stir in the broth, lemon zest, seasoning blend, and cayenne. Cook for 1 minute, or until the mixture is heated through, stirring occasionally.

Add the spinach, tossing with two spoons to lightly coat with the broth mixture. Bring to a simmer, covered, over medium-high heat. Reduce the heat and simmer for 2 to 3 minutes, or until the spinach is slightly wilted, stirring occasionally. Increase the heat to medium-high. Cook for 1 to 2 minutes, or until the spinach is completely wilted and tender, stirring occasionally.

Stir the reserved half-and-half mixture into the spinach mixture. Simmer for 2 to 3 minutes, or until thickened, stirring occasionally.

½ cup fat-free half-and-half

2 tablespoons shredded or grated Parmesan cheese

1½ tablespoons all-purpose flour

1 teaspoon olive oil

2 medium shallots, finely chopped

¼ cup Chicken Broth (page 50) or commercial fat-free, low-sodium chicken broth

1 teaspoon grated lemon zest

½ teaspoon salt-free all-purpose seasoning blend

⅛ teaspoon cayenne (optional)

8 ounces spinach (about 8 cups)

PER SERVING

calories 71	**cholesterol** 2 mg	**protein** 5 g	**dietary exchanges**
total fat 2.0 g	**sodium** 120 mg	**calcium** 133 mg	½ starch
saturated 0.5 g	**carbohydrates** 10 g	**potassium** 356 mg	½ fat
trans 0.0 g	fiber 2 g		
polyunsaturated 0.0 g	sugars 3 g		
monounsaturated 1.0 g			

ORANGE-GLAZED BUTTERNUT SQUASH

Cooking the squash in a nonstick skillet gives it a caramelized crust that heightens its sweetness, which in turn is complemented by a light glaze of orange.

SERVES 4 | ⅔ cup per serving

In a large nonstick skillet, heat the oil over medium heat, swirling to coat the bottom. Cook the squash, covered, for 10 to 12 minutes, or until it is tender and lightly browned, stirring occasionally.

Stir in the orange juice, marmalade, and salt. Cook, uncovered, for 3 minutes, or until most of the liquid is evaporated, stirring occasionally.

2 teaspoons olive oil

1¼ pounds butternut squash, peeled, cut into ¾-inch pieces

2 tablespoons fresh orange juice

2 tablespoons all-fruit orange marmalade

⅛ teaspoon salt

COOK'S TIP ON BUTTERNUT SQUASH If you can't find either bags of precut peeled squash chunks or a small enough single piece of precut squash, buy a whole squash, cut it in half lengthwise, and scoop out and discard the seeds. Peel it and cut it into ¾-inch pieces. Be sure your knife is sharp and be very careful when halving the squash—the skin is quite hard.

PER SERVING

calories 92	**cholesterol** 0 mg	**protein** 1 g	**dietary exchanges**
total fat 2.5 g	**sodium** 78 mg	**calcium** 50 mg	1 starch
saturated 0.5 g	**carbohydrates** 18 g	**potassium** 361 mg	½ fat
trans 0.0 g	fiber 4 g		
polyunsaturated 0.5 g	sugars 8 g		
monounsaturated 1.5 g			

DILLED SUMMER SQUASH

With this recipe, you don't need to buy many ingredients or spend much time in the kitchen to get a colorful and tasty side dish.

SERVES 4 | ¾ cup per serving

In a medium saucepan, bring the water to a boil over high heat. Stir in the remaining ingredients except the oil. Reduce the heat to medium and cook, covered, for 10 minutes, or until the squash is tender. Drain well in a colander. Transfer to a serving bowl.

Add the oil, tossing to coat.

½ cup water

4 medium yellow summer squash, sliced

1 tablespoon finely chopped onion

1 tablespoon snipped fresh dillweed or 1 teaspoon dried, crumbled

¼ teaspoon pepper

1 teaspoon olive oil

PER SERVING

calories 43	**cholesterol** 0 mg	**protein** 2 g	**dietary exchanges**
total fat 1.5 g	**sodium** 5 mg	**calcium** 32 mg	1 vegetable
saturated 0.0 g	**carbohydrates** 7 g	**potassium** 520 mg	½ fat
trans 0.0 g	fiber 2 g		
polyunsaturated 0.5 g	sugars 4 g		
monounsaturated 1.0 g			

SWEET POTATO CASSEROLE

Instead of making the traditional recipe for this southern holiday favorite, give our version a try. It tastes just as good but is much lower in sodium and contains no saturated fat.

SERVES 4 | heaping ½ cup per serving

If using fresh sweet potatoes, pour enough water into a stockpot to cover them. Bring the water to a boil over high heat. Add the sweet potatoes. Return to a boil. Boil for 25 to 30 minutes, or until tender. Using tongs or a slotted spoon, transfer the sweet potatoes to a large bowl of cold water. Soak until cool enough to handle.

Put the sweet potatoes (fresh or canned) in a medium bowl. Mash the sweet potatoes.

Meanwhile, preheat the oven to 375°F. Lightly spray a 1-quart glass casserole dish with cooking spray. Set aside.

Stir the remaining ingredients into the sweet potatoes. Spoon into the casserole dish, gently smoothing the top.

Bake for 25 minutes, or until heated through.

4 medium sweet potatoes or
2 15-ounce cans sweet potatoes, packed without liquid or in water, drained if packed in water

Cooking spray

¼ cup fresh orange juice

2 tablespoons chopped walnuts

¼ teaspoon ground nutmeg

¼ teaspoon brandy flavoring

PER SERVING

calories 144
total fat 2.5 g
 saturated 0.5 g
 trans 0.0 g
 polyunsaturated 1.5 g
 monounsaturated 0.5 g

cholesterol 0 mg
sodium 72 mg
carbohydrates 28 g
 fiber 4 g
 sugars 7 g

protein 3 g
calcium 36 mg
potassium 389 mg

dietary exchanges
 2 starch

BAKED ITALIAN VEGETABLE MÉLANGE

Roasting veggies over high heat retains those delightful concentrated flavors.

SERVES 4 | ½ cup per serving

Preheat the oven to 400°F. Lightly spray a 9-inch pie pan with cooking spray.

In the pie pan, layer as follows: squash, bell pepper, onion, and tomatoes. Sprinkle in order with the red pepper flakes, salt, oregano, basil, and fennel seeds. Lightly spray with cooking spray.

Bake for 25 minutes, or until the vegetables are tender when pierced with a fork. Remove from the oven.

Sprinkle with the parsley and Parmesan. Let stand, covered, for 5 minutes so the flavors blend and the vegetables release their juices.

COOK'S TIP Don't skip the last step. It brings out the flavors while the vegetables "relax" and the juices are released, giving the dish more intensity.

Cooking spray

- 6 ounces yellow summer squash, sliced
- ½ medium green bell pepper, thinly sliced
- ½ large onion, thinly sliced
- 2 medium Italian plum (Roma) tomatoes, cut crosswise into thin slices
- ⅛ teaspoon crushed red pepper flakes
- ⅛ teaspoon salt
- ½ teaspoon dried oregano, crumbled
- ½ teaspoon dried basil, crumbled
- ⅛ teaspoon dried fennel seeds
- 2 tablespoons snipped fresh parsley
- 2 tablespoons shredded or grated Parmesan cheese

PER SERVING

calories 38	**cholesterol** 2 mg	**protein** 2 g	**dietary exchanges**
total fat 1.0 g	**sodium** 120 mg	**calcium** 59 mg	1 vegetable
saturated 0.5 g	**carbohydrates** 6 g	**potassium** 275 mg	
trans 0.0 g	fiber 2 g		
polyunsaturated 0.0 g	sugars 4 g		
monounsaturated 0.0 g			

SAUCES, CONDIMENTS & SEASONINGS

WHITE SAUCE

Whenever you need a basic white sauce, this recipe does the trick. It's also a useful substitute when a casserole recipe calls for a can of condensed creamy soup, which is usually high in sodium.

SERVES 8 | ¼ cup per serving

In a medium saucepan, melt the margarine over medium-low heat, swirling to coat the bottom. Whisk in the flour. Cook for 1 to 2 minutes, whisking occasionally.

Gradually whisk in the milk. Whisk in the lemon juice and pepper. Increase the heat to medium high and bring to a simmer. Simmer for 4 to 5 minutes, whisking constantly. Continue cooking until the sauce has thickened to the desired consistency, whisking constantly.

2 tablespoons light tub margarine

3 tablespoons all-purpose flour

2 cups fat-free milk

1 teaspoon fresh lemon juice

¼ teaspoon pepper, or to taste

WHITE SAUCE
with Parmesan Cheese

Whisk in ¼ cup shredded or grated Parmesan cheese with the lemon juice and pepper for a great sauce to serve over pasta.

WHITE SAUCE
with Dijon Mustard

For a different flavor to go with chicken or fish, whisk in 2 tablespoons Dijon mustard (lowest sodium available) with the lemon juice and pepper.

PER SERVING

calories 42	**cholesterol** 1 mg	**protein** 2 g	**dietary exchanges**
total fat 1.0 g	**sodium** 48 mg	**calcium** 77 mg	½ starch
saturated 0.0 g	**carbohydrates** 5 g	**potassium** 102 mg	
trans 0.0 g	fiber 0 g		
polyunsaturated 0.5 g	sugars 3 g		
monounsaturated 0.5 g			

PER SERVING
WITH PARMESAN CHEESE

calories 52	**cholesterol** 3 mg	**protein** 3 g	**dietary exchanges**
total fat 2.0 g	**sodium** 91 mg	**calcium** 109 mg	½ starch
saturated 0.5 g	**carbohydrates** 6 g	**potassium** 104 mg	
trans 0.0 g	fiber 0 g		
polyunsaturated 0.5 g	sugars 3 g		
monounsaturated 1.0 g			

PER SERVING
WITH DIJON MUSTARD

calories 41	**cholesterol** 1 mg	**protein** 3 g	**dietary exchanges**
total fat 1.5 g	**sodium** 125 mg	**calcium** 80 mg	½ starch
saturated 0.0 g	**carbohydrates** 6 g	**potassium** 109 mg	
trans 0.0 g	fiber 0 g		
polyunsaturated 0.5 g	sugars 3 g		
monounsaturated 0.5 g			

GOURMET MUSHROOM SAUCE

Simple main dishes, such as broiled or grilled steak, pork chops, chicken breasts, or leftover Meat Loaf (page 184), get all dressed up with the addition of this sauce.

SERVES 8 | ¼ cup per serving

In a large nonstick skillet, melt the margarine over medium heat, swirling to coat the bottom. Cook the mushrooms and shallots for 4 to 5 minutes, or until the mushrooms are soft, stirring occasionally.

Sprinkle the flour over the mushroom mixture, stirring to combine.

Gradually add the milk, stirring constantly. Stir in the pepper and garlic powder. Increase the heat to medium high and cook for 4 to 5 minutes, or until the mixture has thickened, stirring occasionally.

Stir in the wine.

2 tablespoons light tub margarine

8 ounces mushrooms, such as button, shiitake, cremini (brown), oyster, or chanterelle, or a combination, sliced

2 medium shallots, finely chopped

3 tablespoons all-purpose flour

2 cups fat-free milk

⅛ teaspoon pepper

⅛ teaspoon garlic powder

1 tablespoon dry white wine (regular or nonalcoholic) or 1 to 2 teaspoons fresh lemon juice

PER SERVING

calories 52
total fat 1.5 g
  saturated 0.0 g
  trans 0.0 g
  polyunsaturated 0.5 g
  monounsaturated 0.5 g

cholesterol 1 mg
sodium 50 mg
carbohydrates 7 g
  fiber 0 g
  sugars 4 g

protein 3 g
calcium 80 mg
potassium 205 mg

dietary exchanges
½ starch

YOGURT DILL SAUCE

Serve this easy sauce over fish, use it as a dip for raw vegetables, or spoon it over sliced cucumbers.

SERVES 4 | ¼ cup per serving

In a small bowl, whisk together all the ingredients. Cover and refrigerate for at least 1 hour before serving.

1 cup fat-free plain yogurt

2 tablespoons snipped fresh dillweed or 2 teaspoons dried, crumbled

2 tablespoons fat-free sour cream

1 teaspoon Dijon mustard (lowest sodium available)

½ teaspoon sugar

½ teaspoon fresh lemon juice

¼ teaspoon pepper

PER SERVING

calories 21	**cholesterol** 1 mg	**protein** 2 g	**dietary exchanges**
total fat 0.0 g	**sodium** 35 mg	**calcium** 62 mg	free
saturated 0.0 g	**carbohydrates** 3 g	**potassium** 80 mg	
trans 0.0 g	fiber 0 g		
polyunsaturated 0.0 g	sugars 3 g		
monounsaturated 0.0 g			

SPAGHETTI SAUCE

Make a batch of this wonderful sauce ahead of time for the best blending of flavors. It will keep in an airtight container in the refrigerator for up to a week, or pour it into a freezer container and freeze it for up to six months.

SERVES 6 | ½ cup per serving

Put the tomato paste in a medium saucepan. Whisk in the water, 1 cup at a time.

Whisk in the remaining ingredients. Bring to a boil over medium-high heat. Reduce the heat and simmer, covered, for 30 minutes, or until the desired consistency, stirring occasionally.

2 6-ounce cans no-salt-added tomato paste

2 cups water

¼ cup finely chopped onion

2 medium garlic cloves, minced

1 teaspoon dried basil, crumbled

1 teaspoon dried oregano, crumbled

½ teaspoon dried thyme, crumbled

½ teaspoon sugar

⅛ teaspoon pepper

⅛ teaspoon crushed red pepper flakes (optional)

PER SERVING

calories 54
total fat 0.5 g
  saturated 0.0 g
  trans 0.0 g
  polyunsaturated 0.0 g
  monounsaturated 0.0 g

cholesterol 0 mg
sodium 59 mg
carbohydrates 12 g
  fiber 3 g
  sugars 8 g

protein 3 g
calcium 36 mg
potassium 603 mg

dietary exchanges
2 vegetable

BARBECUE SAUCE

After trying our healthful version of barbecue sauce, you'll wonder why you ever bought the bottled kind.

MAKES 4 CUPS | ¼ cup per serving

In a large saucepan, whisk together all the ingredients. Bring to a boil over high heat. Reduce the heat and simmer for 20 minutes, whisking occasionally. Refrigerate the sauce in a jar with a tight-fitting lid for up to one month or freeze it in an airtight freezer container for up to six months.

- 2 cups water
- 2 6-ounce cans no-salt-added tomato paste
- ½ cup no-salt-added ketchup
- ¼ cup firmly packed dark brown sugar
- ¼ cup chopped onion
- 2 tablespoons Chili Powder (page 277) or no-salt-added chili powder
- 2 tablespoons fresh lemon juice
- 2 tablespoons cider vinegar
- 2 tablespoons canola or corn oil
- 1 tablespoon snipped fresh parsley
- 1 teaspoon dry mustard
- 1 teaspoon paprika
- 1 medium garlic clove, minced
- ⅛ teaspoon pepper
- Dash of red hot-pepper sauce (optional)

PER SERVING

calories 60
total fat 2.0 g
  saturated 0.0 g
  trans 0.0 g
  polyunsaturated 0.5 g
  monounsaturated 1.0 g

cholesterol 0 mg
sodium 25 mg
carbohydrates 10 g
  fiber 1 g
  sugars 8 g

protein 1 g
calcium 18 mg
potassium 283 mg

dietary exchanges
  ½ other carbohydrate
  ½ fat

STRAWBERRY ORANGE SAUCE

Easy to make, this topping turns ordinary fat-free vanilla yogurt or ice cream into something special. Instead of using syrup on our Pancakes (page 290), try this as a less-sugary, healthier alternative.

MAKES 3 CUPS | ¼ cup per serving

In a small saucepan, heat the liqueur and orange juice over medium heat.

Stir in 1¾ cups strawberries. Cook for 2 minutes, stirring frequently.

Stir in the sugar. Cook for 2 to 3 minutes, or until the berries soften. Remove from the heat.

Stir in the remaining 1¾ cups strawberries. Serve hot or pour into a small airtight container and refrigerate until ready to serve.

1 tablespoon orange-flavored liqueur and 1 tablespoon fresh orange juice, or 2 tablespoons fresh orange juice

1¾ cups strawberries and 1¾ cups strawberries (about 1 quart total), all hulled and sliced lengthwise, divided use

1 tablespoon sugar

CINNAMON BLUEBERRY SAUCE

Substitute fresh blueberries for the strawberries and use 2 tablespoons of fresh orange juice. Add ½ teaspoon ground cinnamon when stirring in the sugar.

PER SERVING

calories 33	**cholesterol** 0 mg	**protein** 0 g	**dietary exchanges**
total fat 0.0 g	**sodium** 1 mg	**calcium** 11 mg	½ fruit
saturated 0.0 g	**carbohydrates** 7 g	**potassium** 102 mg	
trans 0.0 g	fiber 1 g		
polyunsaturated 0.0 g	sugars 5 g		
monounsaturated 0.0 g			

PER SERVING
CINNAMON BLUEBERRY SAUCE

calories 45	**cholesterol** 0 mg	**protein** 1 g	**dietary exchanges**
total fat 0.0 g	**sodium** 1 mg	**calcium** 6 mg	1 fruit
saturated 0.0 g	**carbohydrates** 11 g	**potassium** 58 mg	
trans 0.0 g	fiber 2 g		
polyunsaturated 0.0 g	sugars 8 g		
monounsaturated 0.0 g			

FRESH SPINACH AND BASIL PESTO

Fresh spinach adds a new dimension to basil-based pesto. Try the pesto as a topping for chicken, fish, or pasta.

SERVES 4 | 2 tablespoons per serving

With the food processor running, drop the garlic cloves into the food chute and process for 5 seconds. Add the basil, spinach, Parmesan, and pine nuts to the processor bowl. Process for 20 to 30 seconds, or until smooth, scraping the side once.

With the processor running, slowly pour 1 tablespoon water, the lemon juice, and oil through the food chute. Process for 10 seconds, or until well blended. While continuing to process, gradually add more water if needed for the desired consistency. Serve at room temperature or refrigerate in an airtight container for two to three days. Return refrigerated pesto to room temperature before serving, if desired.

- 3 medium garlic cloves
- 1 cup packed fresh basil (about 2½ ounces before removing stems)
- 1 cup packed baby spinach (about 2 ounces)
- 3 tablespoons shredded or grated Parmesan cheese
- 1 tablespoon pine nuts
- 1 tablespoon water (plus more as needed)
- 2 teaspoons fresh lemon juice
- 2 teaspoons olive oil (extra virgin preferred)

PER SERVING

calories 53	**cholesterol** 3 mg	**protein** 3 g	**dietary exchanges**
total fat 4.5 g	**sodium** 71 mg	**calcium** 78 mg	1 fat
saturated 1.0 g	**carbohydrates** 2 g	**potassium** 100 mg	
trans 0.0 g	fiber 1 g		
polyunsaturated 0.5 g	sugars 0 g		
monounsaturated 2.5 g			

ROASTED TOMATO CHIPOTLE SALSA

Spice up lean grilled hamburgers, chicken breasts, or pork tenderloin with this wonderful salsa, which gets its smoky flavor from the chipotle chile. Regulate the heat from mild to spicy by the amount of chipotle you add.

SERVES 4 | 3 tablespoons per serving

Preheat the oven to 400°F. Lightly spray a large baking sheet with cooking spray.

Put the tomato quarters, shallot, and garlic on the baking sheet (the garlic will be easier to peel after roasting).

Roast for 20 minutes, or until the garlic is light golden brown.

Peel the tomato and garlic, discarding the skins.

In a food processor or blender, process all the ingredients for 10 to 15 seconds, or until the desired consistency. Serve or pour into a small airtight container and refrigerate for up to four days.

Cooking spray
- 1 large tomato, quartered
- 1 large whole shallot or one 1½-inch-thick slice of red onion, quartered
- 2 medium garlic cloves, unpeeled
- 1 tablespoon whole cilantro leaves
- 1 to 2 teaspoons fresh lime juice
- ½ to 2 teaspoons chopped canned chipotle pepper in adobo sauce or 1 teaspoon chopped fresh jalapeño

PER SERVING

calories 16
total fat 0.0 g
  saturated 0.0 g
  trans 0.0 g
  polyunsaturated 0.0 g
  monounsaturated 0.0 g

cholesterol 0 mg
sodium 25 mg
carbohydrates 3 g
  fiber 1 g
  sugars 1 g

protein 1 g
calcium 9 mg
potassium 130 mg

dietary exchanges
free

PINEAPPLE-KIWI SALSA

Sweet and spicy, this fruit salsa is a refreshing accompaniment to grilled chicken, pork, fish, or shrimp. It is also great as a quick, healthy snack when served on apple or pear slices or warm whole-wheat pita triangles.

MAKES 2 CUPS | ¼ cup per serving

In a medium bowl, gently stir together all the ingredients. Let stand at room temperature for 10 to 15 minutes before serving so the flavors blend. Cover any leftovers and refrigerate for use the next day.

¾ cup finely chopped fresh pineapple

2 medium kiwifruit, peeled and chopped

2 medium strawberries, hulled and chopped

3 tablespoons snipped fresh cilantro

2 tablespoons chopped red onion

½ to 1 medium fresh jalapeño, seeds and ribs discarded, minced

1 teaspoon grated lime zest

1 tablespoon fresh lime juice

1 teaspoon snipped fresh mint

½ teaspoon honey

PER SERVING

calories 12
total fat 0.0 g
  saturated 0.0 g
  trans 0.0 g
  polyunsaturated 0.0 g
  monounsaturated 0.0 g

cholesterol 0 mg
sodium 1 mg
carbohydrates 3 g
  fiber 1 g
  sugars 2 g

protein 0 g
calcium 6 mg
potassium 46 mg

dietary exchanges
free

APPLE-GINGER CHUTNEY

Apples cooked in orange juice and flavored with fresh ginger and spices—the combination smells as delicious as it tastes! Serve the chutney with roast pork, chicken, or turkey.

SERVES 7 | ¼ cup per serving

Lightly spray a small saucepan with cooking spray. Cook the onion and garlic over medium heat for about 3 minutes, or until the onion just softens, stirring frequently.

Stir in the remaining ingredients. Bring to a simmer. Reduce the heat and simmer for 20 minutes, or until the apples are tender and the liquids have reduced to 1 to 2 tablespoons, stirring occasionally. Serve warm or transfer to an airtight container and refrigerate for about 1 hour to serve chilled. Refrigerate any leftovers for up to three days.

Cooking spray

- ¼ cup chopped red onion
- 1 medium garlic clove, minced
- 2 medium Granny Smith apples, peeled and chopped
- ¼ cup fresh orange juice
- 1 tablespoon plus 1 teaspoon light brown sugar
- 2 teaspoons minced peeled gingerroot
- ¼ teaspoon ground allspice
- ⅛ teaspoon ground cloves
- ⅛ teaspoon pepper

PER SERVING

calories 20	**cholesterol** 0 mg	**protein** 0 g	**dietary exchanges**
total fat 0.0 g	**sodium** 1 mg	**calcium** 4 mg	free
saturated 0.0 g	**carbohydrates** 5 g	**potassium** 38 mg	
trans 0.0 g	fiber 0 g		
polyunsaturated 0.0 g	sugars 4 g		
monounsaturated 0.0 g			

EASY DILL PICKLES

Even if you've never made pickles before, don't hesitate to try this recipe. It is so easy! Just let the cucumbers simmer in a flavorful liquid, then cool and refrigerate them. The flavor of these pickles really brightens lean grilled burgers or your favorite potato salad or tuna salad recipe.

MAKES 4 CUPS | ¼ cup per serving

With a knife or crinkle cutter, cut the cucumbers crosswise into ¼-inch slices. You should have about 4 cups. Line a colander with two or three paper towels. Put the cucumbers in the colander, cover with additional paper towels, and set a plate on top to slightly weigh the cucumbers down (this will help remove any excess moisture). Let stand for 5 to 10 minutes.

In a large saucepan, bring the remaining ingredients to a boil over high heat. Reduce the heat to medium and stir in the cucumbers. Cook for 3 minutes, or until tender-crisp, stirring occasionally. Remove from the heat and let cool for 15 minutes. Transfer to an airtight container large enough to hold the cucumbers and liquid (a clean large pickle jar works well) and refrigerate for at least 4 hours before serving. The pickles will keep in the refrigerator for up to two weeks.

1 pound pickling, or Kirby, cucumbers (about 4), unpeeled
1 cup water
¾ cup cider vinegar
1 tablespoon dill seeds
1 tablespoon whole pickling spices
1 tablespoon sugar
2 medium garlic cloves
4 or 5 sprigs of fresh dillweed (optional)

COOK'S TIP ON PICKLING, OR KIRBY, CUCUMBERS As its name tells you, this small cucumber variety is primarily used for pickles. It's also used as a garnish in many Asian dishes and can be substituted for the more common cucumber. Pickling cucumbers have thin skin, are crisp, and have very small seeds. Many groceries carry them regularly, or you can look for them at a local farmers' market or Asian grocery store. A great alternative is the English, or hothouse, cucumber (see Cook's Tip on English Cucumbers, page 76). You can also pickle the common cucumber.

COOK'S TIP ON PICKLING SPICES You'll find pickling spices in the spice section of the grocery. Commercial brands of this aromatic mix of spices vary but can include allspice, cinnamon, mustard seeds, coriander seeds, ginger, bay leaves, chiles, pepper, cloves, cardamom, and mace. Use 1 teaspoon to 1 tablespoon of the mixture in marinades, water for cooking shrimp, or soups and stews. Use kitchen twine to tie the spices in a small piece of cheesecloth so you can remove them easily.

PER SERVING

calories 11	**cholesterol** 0 mg	**protein** 0 g	**dietary exchanges**
total fat 0.0 g	**sodium** 1 mg	**calcium** 17 mg	free
saturated 0.0 g	**carbohydrates** 2 g	**potassium** 57 mg	
trans 0.0 g	fiber 1 g		
polyunsaturated 0.0 g	sugars 1 g		
monounsaturated 0.0 g			

SWEET BREAD-AND-BUTTER PICKLES

These quick-fix pickles have the traditional flavor you expect but only 1 milligram of sodium, a tremendous saving compared to commercial pickles of the same variety.

MAKES 4 CUPS | ¼ cup per serving

With a knife or crinkle cutter, cut the cucumbers crosswise into ¼-inch slices. You should have about 4 cups. Line a colander with two or three paper towels. Put the cucumbers and onion in the colander, cover with additional paper towels, and set a plate on top to slightly weigh the cucumber mixture down (this will help remove any excess moisture). Let stand for 5 to 10 minutes.

In a large saucepan, bring the remaining ingredients to a boil over high heat. Reduce the heat to medium and stir in the cucumbers and onion. Cook for 3 minutes, or until tender-crisp, stirring occasionally. Remove from the heat and let cool for 15 minutes. Transfer to an airtight container large enough to hold the cucumber mixture and liquid (a clean large pickle jar works well) and refrigerate for at least 4 hours before serving. The pickles will keep in the refrigerator for up to two weeks.

1 pound pickling, or Kirby, cucumbers (about 4), unpeeled
1 medium onion, sliced
1 cup water
¾ cup cider vinegar
½ cup sugar
1 teaspoon pink peppercorns (optional)
½ teaspoon mustard seeds
¼ teaspoon turmeric

SWEET PICKLE RELISH

Finely chop the cucumbers and onion, and add 1 finely chopped medium green or red bell pepper. Bring all the ingredients to a simmer over medium-high heat. Reduce the heat and simmer for 10 to 15 minutes, or until the relish is thickened, stirring occasionally. Store as directed on page 274.

COOK'S TIP ON PINK PEPPERCORNS These dried berries from the Baies rose plant are not true peppercorns, but are peppery in taste and beautiful in color. Find them in gourmet shops or upscale grocery stores.

PER SERVING

calories 33	**cholesterol** 0 mg	**protein** 0 g	**dietary exchanges**
total fat 0.0 g	**sodium** 1 mg	**calcium** 10 mg	½ other carbohydrate
saturated 0.0 g	**carbohydrates** 8 g	**potassium** 62 mg	
trans 0.0 g	fiber 1 g		
polyunsaturated 0.0 g	sugars 7 g		
monounsaturated 0.0 g			

PER SERVING
SWEET PICKLE RELISH

calories 35	**cholesterol** 0 mg	**protein** 0 g	**dietary exchanges**
total fat 0.0 g	**sodium** 2 mg	**calcium** 11 mg	½ other carbohydrate
saturated 0.0 g	**carbohydrates** 8 g	**potassium** 75 mg	
trans 0.0 g	fiber 1 g		
polyunsaturated 0.0 g	sugars 7 g		
monounsaturated 0.0 g			

CHILI SAUCE

Add some zing to your food, but without the sodium usually found in bottled chili sauce. Drizzle this chili sauce on Spicy Baked Fish (page 103) or use it to make shrimp cocktail.

MAKES 3 CUPS | 2 tablespoons per serving

In a large saucepan, whisk together all the ingredients. Bring to a boil over high heat, whisking frequently. Reduce the heat and simmer for 1 hour 30 minutes, or until reduced by half, to about 3 cups, whisking occasionally. Refrigerate in a jar with a tight-fitting lid for up to one month or freeze in an airtight freezer container for up to six months.

2 16-ounce cans no-salt-added tomato sauce

½ cup sugar

½ cup chopped onion

1 medium rib of celery, chopped

½ medium green bell pepper, chopped

½ cup cider vinegar

2 tablespoons light tub margarine

1 tablespoon fresh lemon juice

1 teaspoon light brown sugar

1 teaspoon light molasses

¼ teaspoon red hot-pepper sauce

⅛ teaspoon ground cloves

⅛ teaspoon ground cinnamon

⅛ teaspoon pepper

⅛ teaspoon dried basil, crumbled

⅛ teaspoon dried tarragon, crumbled

PER SERVING

calories 36	**cholesterol** 0 mg	**protein** 1 g	**dietary exchanges**
total fat 0.5 g	**sodium** 14 mg	**calcium** 9 mg	½ other carbohydrate
saturated 0.0 g	**carbohydrates** 8 g	**potassium** 165 mg	
trans 0.0 g	fiber 1 g		
polyunsaturated 0.0 g	sugars 6 g		
monounsaturated 0.0 g			

CHILI POWDER

Try this in your own favorite chili recipe, our Chili (page 190), or Eggplant Mexicana (page 244).

MAKES ¼ CUP | 1 teaspoon per serving

In a small bowl, stir together all the ingredients. Transfer to a jar with a tight-fitting lid and store in a cool, dark, dry place for up to six months.

3 tablespoons paprika

2 teaspoons dried oregano, crumbled

1 teaspoon ground cumin

1 teaspoon turmeric

1 teaspoon garlic powder

¼ teaspoon cayenne

PER SERVING

calories 8	**cholesterol** 0 mg	**protein** 0 g	**dietary exchanges**
total fat 0.5 g	**sodium** 1 mg	**calcium** 8 mg	free
saturated 0.0 g	**carbohydrates** 1 g	**potassium** 52 mg	
trans 0.0 g	fiber 1 g		
polyunsaturated 0.0 g	sugars 0 g		
monounsaturated 0.0 g			

CREOLE SEASONING

Use this spicy mix in Zesty Oven-Fried Potatoes (page 250) and any other recipes that call for Creole or Cajun seasoning blends.

MAKES 2 TABLESPOONS | ½ teaspoon per serving

In a small bowl, stir together all the ingredients. Transfer to a jar with a tight-fitting lid and store in a cool, dark, dry place for up to six months.

- 1 teaspoon Chili Powder (page 277) or no-salt-added chili powder
- 1 teaspoon paprika
- 1 teaspoon ground cumin
- 1 teaspoon dried thyme, crumbled
- ½ teaspoon garlic powder
- ½ teaspoon onion powder
- ½ teaspoon pepper

PER SERVING

calories 3	**cholesterol** 0 mg	**protein** 0 g	**dietary exchanges** free
total fat 0.0 g	**sodium** 1 mg	**calcium** 4 mg	
saturated 0.0 g	**carbohydrates** 1 g	**potassium** 16 mg	
trans 0.0 g	fiber 0 g		
polyunsaturated 0.0 g	sugars 0 g		
monounsaturated 0.0 g			

BREADS & BREAKFAST DISHES

ROSEMARY RYE BREAD

It won't take you long to do the actual preparation for this aromatic bread. During its resting and baking times, you can take a walk, fix dinner, or just relax.

SERVES 16 | 1 slice per serving

Lightly spray a baking sheet with the olive oil spray. Set aside.

In a large bowl, stir together 1¼ cups all-purpose flour and the rye flour, gluten flour, rosemary, caraway seeds, oil, yeast, and salt.

Add the water, stirring for about 30 seconds.

Gradually add some of the remaining 1 cup all-purpose flour, beating with a spoon after each addition, until the dough starts to pull away from the side of the bowl. Add more flour if necessary to make the dough stiff enough to handle.

Lightly flour a flat surface. Turn out the dough. Knead for 6 to 7 minutes, gradually adding enough of the remaining flour to make the dough smooth and elastic. (The dough shouldn't be dry or stick to the surface. You may not need the additional flour, or you may need up to ½ cup more if the dough is too sticky.) Leave the dough on the work surface. Cover the dough with a slightly damp dish towel. Let rest for 10 minutes.

Olive oil spray
1¼ cups all-purpose flour and 1 cup all-purpose flour (plus more as needed), divided use
¾ cup rye flour
1 tablespoon gluten flour
1 tablespoon fresh rosemary, chopped, or 1 teaspoon dried, crushed
1 tablespoon caraway seeds
1 tablespoon olive oil
2 teaspoons fast-rising yeast
½ teaspoon salt
1¼ cups warm water (120°F to 130°F)

Shape the dough into a 9 x 5-inch oval loaf. Put the loaf on the baking sheet and flatten slightly with your hands. Using a serrated knife, cut a few widthwise slashes about 3 inches long and ½ inch deep in the top of the loaf. Cover with a dry dish towel and let rise in a warm, draft-free place (about 85°F) for 30 to 45 minutes, or until doubled in bulk. Near the end of the rising cycle, preheat the oven to 375°F.

Bake for 35 to 40 minutes, or until the bread registers 190°F on an instant-read thermometer or sounds hollow when rapped with your knuckles. Turn out onto a cooling rack and let cool for 15 minutes before slicing.

COOK'S TIP To make Rosemary Rye Bread using a bread machine, follow the directions on page 282.

PER SERVING

calories 93	**cholesterol** 0 mg	**protein** 3 g	**dietary exchanges**
total fat 1.0 g	**sodium** 74 mg	**calcium** 8 mg	1 starch
saturated 0.0 g	**carbohydrates** 18 g	**potassium** 52 mg	
trans 0.0 g	fiber 2 g		
polyunsaturated 0.0 g	sugars 0 g		
monounsaturated 0.5 g			

ROSEMARY RYE BREAD
BREAD MACHINE INSTRUCTIONS

Follow the manufacturer's instructions for the quick baking cycle. If you prefer, use the quick dough cycle, shape the loaf by hand when the dough is ready, and bake the bread in the oven as directed on page 281.

SERVES 12, 18, OR 24 | 1 slice per serving

	1-POUND MACHINE (12 servings)	1½-POUND MACHINE (18 servings)	2-POUND MACHINE (24 servings)
Water (tap)	¾ cup	1¼ cups	1½ cups
Olive oil	1 tablespoon	1½ tablespoons	2 tablespoons
All-purpose flour	1½ cups	2¼ cups	3 cups
Rye flour	½ cup	¾ cup	1 cup
Gluten flour	2 teaspoons	1 tablespoon	1 tablespoon plus 1 teaspoon
Fresh rosemary leaves, chopped (or dried rosemary, crushed)	2 teaspoons / ½ teaspoon	1 tablespoon / 1 teaspoon	1 tablespoon plus 1 teaspoon / 1½ teaspoons
Caraway seeds	2 teaspoons	1 tablespoon	1 tablespoon plus 1 teaspoon
Salt	¼ teaspoon	½ teaspoon	½ teaspoon
Fast-rising yeast	1 teaspoon	1½ teaspoons	2 teaspoons

PER SERVING

calories 86
total fat 1.5 g
  saturated 0.0 g
  trans 0.0 g
  polyunsaturated 0.0 g
  monounsaturated 1.0 g

cholesterol 0 mg
sodium 50 mg
carbohydrates 16 g
  fiber 1 g
  sugars 0 g

protein 2 g
calcium 7 mg
potassium 44 mg

dietary exchanges
1 starch

WHOLE-WHEAT BREAD

Get back to basics, and take pleasure in baking your own nourishing bread.

SERVES 12, 18, OR 24 | 1 slice per serving

	1-POUND MACHINE (12 servings)	1½-POUND MACHINE (18 servings)	2-POUND MACHINE (24 servings)
Fat-free milk	⅔ cup	¾ cup plus 2 tablespoons	1¼ cups plus 1 tablespoon
Water	2 tablespoons	3 tablespoons	¼ cup
Canola or corn oil	2¼ teaspoons	1 tablespoon	1½ tablespoons
All-purpose flour	1 cup	1½ cups	2 cups
Whole-wheat flour	1 cup	1½ cups	2 cups
Gluten flour	1 tablespoon	1½ tablespoons	2 tablespoons
Molasses	1 tablespoon	1½ tablespoons	2 tablespoons
Active dry yeast	2 teaspoons	2½ teaspoons	1 tablespoon

Put the ingredients in the bread machine container in the order recommended by the manufacturer. Select the whole-grain or basic/white bread cycle. Proceed as directed by the manufacturer. When the bread is done, let cool on a cooling rack before slicing.

PER SERVING

calories 93	**cholesterol** 0 mg	**protein** 3 g	**dietary exchanges**
total fat 1.0 g	**sodium** 7 mg	**calcium** 26 mg	1 starch
saturated 0.0 g	**carbohydrates** 18 g	**potassium** 108 mg	
trans 0.0 g	fiber 2 g		
polyunsaturated 0.5 g	sugars 2 g		
monounsaturated 0.5 g			

OATMEAL BANANA BREAKFAST BREAD

Banana, cranberries, and orange zest give this bread a lively flavor that will get your day off to just the right start.

SERVES 16 | 1 slice per serving

Preheat the oven to 350°F. Lightly spray an 8½ x 4½ x 2½-inch loaf pan with cooking spray. Set aside.

In a medium bowl, stir together the milk, ½ cup oatmeal, the brown sugar, banana, dried fruit, egg substitute, oil, and orange zest.

In another medium bowl, stir together the flour, oat bran, baking powder, cinnamon, and baking soda. Add to the milk mixture, stirring just until the batter is moistened but no flour is visible. Don't overmix; the batter should be slightly lumpy. Spoon into the pan, gently smoothing the top. Sprinkle with the remaining 1 tablespoon oatmeal.

Bake for 45 to 50 minutes, or until a wooden toothpick inserted in the center comes out clean. Turn out onto a cooling rack and let cool for at least 10 minutes before slicing.

Cooking spray

¾ cup fat-free milk

½ cup uncooked quick-cooking oatmeal and 1 tablespoon uncooked quick-cooking oatmeal, divided use

½ cup firmly packed light brown sugar

1 medium banana, mashed

½ cup dried fruit, such as cranberries, raisins, or mixed bits

¼ cup egg substitute or 1 large egg

2 tablespoons canola or corn oil

1½ to 2 teaspoons grated orange zest or ½ teaspoon dried orange peel

1½ cups all-purpose flour

½ cup uncooked oat bran

2 teaspoons baking powder

1 to 1½ teaspoons ground cinnamon

¼ teaspoon baking soda

PER SERVING

calories 128	**cholesterol** 0 mg	**protein** 3 g	**dietary exchanges**
total fat 2.5 g	**sodium** 85 mg	**calcium** 61 mg	1½ starch
saturated 0.0 g	**carbohydrates** 25 g	**potassium** 120 mg	½ fat
trans 0.0 g	fiber 2 g		
polyunsaturated 0.5 g	sugars 11 g		
monounsaturated 1.0 g			

BLUEBERRY MUFFINS

Lemon-scented muffins with plump blueberries really hit the spot for breakfast or an afternoon snack.

SERVES 12 | 1 muffin per serving

Preheat the oven to 400°F. Lightly spray a 12-cup muffin pan with cooking spray or line with paper bake cups. Set aside.

In a large bowl, stir together the flour, ⅓ cup sugar, and the baking powder.

In a small bowl, whisk together the milk, egg substitute, applesauce, oil, and lemon zest. Pour into the flour mixture, stirring until the batter is just moistened but no flour is visible. Don't overmix; the batter should be slightly lumpy.

With a rubber scraper, carefully fold in the blueberries. Pour about ¼ cup batter into each muffin cup. Sprinkle with the remaining 1 teaspoon sugar.

Bake for 20 to 22 minutes, or until a wooden toothpick inserted in the center of a muffin comes out clean.

Cooking spray (if not using paper bake cups)

1¾ cups all-purpose flour

⅓ cup sugar and 1 teaspoon sugar, divided use

2½ teaspoons baking powder

½ cup fat-free milk

¼ cup egg substitute or 2 large egg whites

¼ cup unsweetened applesauce

1 tablespoon canola or corn oil

1 teaspoon grated lemon zest

1 cup fresh or frozen blueberries (don't thaw if frozen)

PER SERVING

calories 115	**cholesterol** 0 mg	**protein** 3 g	**dietary exchanges**
total fat 1.5 g	**sodium** 99 mg	**calcium** 68 mg	1½ starch
saturated 0.0 g	**carbohydrates** 23 g	**potassium** 56 mg	
trans 0.0 g	fiber 1 g		
polyunsaturated 0.5 g	sugars 8 g		
monounsaturated 1.0 g			

CORN MUFFINS

Homemade corn muffins make mealtime special. Try them with Lima Bean Soup with Ham Bits and Crisp Sage (page 70) or Pecan-Crusted Catfish with Zesty Tartar Sauce (page 106). Any leftover muffins are super for a grab-and-go snack.

SERVES 12 | 1 muffin per serving

Cooking spray
- 1 cup all-purpose flour
- ¾ cup yellow or white cornmeal
- 2 teaspoons baking powder
- 1 cup fat-free milk
- ¼ cup egg substitute or 1 large egg
- 1 tablespoon canola or corn oil
- 1 tablespoon light tub margarine, melted

Preheat the oven to 425°F. Lightly spray a 12-cup muffin pan with cooking spray. Set aside.

In a large bowl, stir together the flour, cornmeal, and baking powder.

In a small bowl, whisk together the remaining ingredients. Pour all at once into the flour mixture, stirring until the batter is just moistened but no flour is visible. Don't overmix; the batter should be slightly lumpy. Pour about ¼ cup batter into each muffin cup.

Bake for 15 to 20 minutes, or until a wooden toothpick inserted in the center of a muffin comes out clean. Turn out onto a cooling rack.

CORN BREAD

SERVES 12 | 1 square per serving

Lightly spray an 8-inch square baking pan with cooking spray. Pour in the batter. Bake for 20 to 25 minutes, or until a wooden toothpick inserted in the center comes out clean. Turn out onto a cooling rack. Let cool and cut into squares.

MEXICAN CORN MUFFINS

SERVES 12 | 1 muffin per serving

To the milk mixture, stir in 1 cup no-salt-added canned or frozen whole-kernel corn, drained if canned or thawed if frozen; ½ cup low-fat-shredded Cheddar cheese; 2 tablespoons canned mild green chiles, drained; and 1 teaspoon Chili Powder (page 277) or no-salt-added chili powder. Continue with the recipe as directed on page 286.

PER SERVING

calories 92	**cholesterol** 0 mg	**protein** 3 g	**dietary exchanges**
total fat 2.0 g	**sodium** 94 mg	**calcium** 69 mg	1 starch
saturated 0.0 g	**carbohydrates** 16 g	**potassium** 65 mg	
trans 0.0 g	fiber 1 g		
polyunsaturated 0.5 g	sugars 1 g		
monounsaturated 1.0 g			

PER SERVING
MEXICAN CORN MUFFINS

calories 115	**cholesterol** 1 mg	**protein** 5 g	**dietary exchanges**
total fat 2.5 g	**sodium** 132 mg	**calcium** 92 mg	1½ starch
saturated 0.5 g	**carbohydrates** 20 g	**potassium** 105 mg	
trans 0.0 g	fiber 1 g		
polyunsaturated 0.5 g	sugars 2 g		
monounsaturated 1.0 g			

OAT BRAN AND YOGURT MUFFINS

These muffins boast more nutrition than a high-calorie snack bar. Pack two muffins in your lunchbox, and share your heart-healthy treat with a friend.

SERVES 12 | 1 muffin per serving

Preheat the oven to 425°F. Lightly spray a 12-cup muffin pan with cooking spray or line with paper bake cups. Set aside.

In a large bowl, stir together the flours, oat bran, raisins, sugar, baking powder, and baking soda.

In a small bowl, whisk together the yogurt, egg substitute, and oil. Pour into the flour mixture, stirring until the batter is just moistened but no flour is visible. Don't overmix; the batter should be slightly lumpy. Pour about ¼ cup batter into each muffin cup.

Bake for 16 to 18 minutes, or until a wooden toothpick inserted in the center of a muffin comes out clean.

Cooking spray (if not using paper bake cups)
¾ cup all-purpose flour
½ cup whole-wheat flour
½ cup uncooked oat bran
½ cup raisins
⅓ cup sugar
2 teaspoons baking powder
¼ teaspoon baking soda
1 cup fat-free plain yogurt
¼ cup egg substitute or 1 large egg
1 tablespoon canola or corn oil

COOK'S TIP ON PAPER BAKE CUPS Let the muffins cool completely before removing the paper bake cups. This will keep the paper from sticking and pulling off part of the muffin.

PER SERVING

calories 122	**cholesterol** 0 mg	**protein** 4 g	**dietary exchanges**
total fat 1.5 g	**sodium** 120 mg	**calcium** 91 mg	1½ starch
saturated 0.0 g	**carbohydrates** 25 g	**potassium** 162 mg	
trans 0.0 g	fiber 2 g		
polyunsaturated 0.5 g	sugars 11 g		
monounsaturated 1.0 g			

BERRY-BUTTERMILK COFFEE CAKE

The raspberries or blueberries peek through the top of this coffee cake, giving a hint of what's inside.

SERVES 10 | 1 piece per serving

Preheat the oven to 350°F. Lightly spray an 8-inch round metal cake pan with cooking spray. Set aside.

In a large bowl, whisk together the flours, baking powder, and baking soda.

In a medium bowl, whisk together the buttermilk, sugar, oil, egg, lemon zest, and vanilla until smooth. Pour into the flour mixture, stirring until the batter is just moistened but no flour is visible.

Spoon half the batter into the pan, spreading to cover the bottom. Sprinkle with the berries. Spoon the remaining batter over the berries, leaving some of them uncovered.

Bake for 35 to 40 minutes, or until a wooden toothpick inserted in the center comes out clean. Transfer the pan to a cooling rack. Let cool for 10 minutes. Turn the coffee cake out onto a cooling rack and let cool completely, about 1 hour. Dust the coffee cake with confectioners' sugar.

Cooking spray
- 1 cup whole-wheat flour
- ½ cup all-purpose flour
- 1½ teaspoons baking powder
- ½ teaspoon baking soda
- ¾ cup low-fat buttermilk
- ⅔ cup sugar
- ¼ cup canola or corn oil
- 1 large egg
- 2 teaspoons grated lemon zest
- 1 teaspoon vanilla extract
- 1 cup fresh or frozen unsweetened raspberries or fresh or frozen blueberries (don't thaw if frozen)
Confectioners' sugar for dusting

PER SERVING

calories 188	**cholesterol** 22 mg	**protein** 4 g	**dietary exchanges**
total fat 6.5 g	**sodium** 150 mg	**calcium** 69 mg	2 other carbohydrate
saturated 0.5 g	**carbohydrates** 30 g	**potassium** 110 mg	1½ fat
trans 0.0 g	fiber 3 g		
polyunsaturated 2.0 g	sugars 15 g		
monounsaturated 4.0 g			

PANCAKES

Whether you serve these pancakes for breakfast, brunch, lunch, or dinner, they'll soon become a family favorite.

SERVES 4 | 2 4-inch pancakes per serving

Preheat the oven to 200°F.

In a medium bowl, stir together the flour, sugar, baking powder, and cinnamon.

In a small bowl, whisk together the remaining ingredients. Pour into the flour mixture, gently whisking until the batter is just moistened but no flour is visible. Don't overmix; the batter should be slightly lumpy.

Heat a nonstick griddle over medium heat. Test the temperature by sprinkling a few drops of water on the griddle. If the water evaporates quickly, the griddle is ready. Spoon ¼ cup batter onto the griddle for each pancake, making 4 pancakes (about half the batter will remain). Cook for 2 to 3 minutes, or until the tops are bubbly and the edges are dry. Turn over. Cook for 2 minutes, or until the bottoms are golden brown. Transfer the pancakes to a plate. Put in the oven to keep warm. Repeat with the remaining batter.

1 cup all-purpose flour

2 tablespoons sugar

2 teaspoons baking powder

⅛ teaspoon ground cinnamon

¾ cup plus 2 tablespoons fat-free milk

¼ cup egg substitute or 1 large egg

2 teaspoons canola or corn oil

¼ teaspoon vanilla extract

BLUEBERRY PANCAKES

Add ½ cup fresh or frozen blueberries (don't thaw) to the batter after combining the pancake ingredients.

COOK'S TIP ON BLUEBERRIES When selecting blueberries, an excellent source of fiber, look for plump, firm berries with a powdery coating. That protective shield preserves moisture and keeps them fresh longer than most other berries. Choose dark blue berries for eating raw; the reddish ones are fine for cooking but are quite tart. Blueberries freeze well. Arrange the unwashed berries in a single layer on a baking sheet so they don't touch, let them freeze solid, then put them in an airtight plastic freezer bag. Just before use, rinse the frozen berries, but don't thaw them or they will bleed on your hands and color the food they touch.

PER SERVING

calories 185	**cholesterol** 1 mg	**protein** 7 g	**dietary exchanges**
total fat 2.5 g	**sodium** 254 mg	**calcium** 198 mg	2 starch
saturated 0.0 g	**carbohydrates** 33 g	**potassium** 139 mg	
trans 0.0 g	fiber 1 g		
polyunsaturated 1.0 g	sugars 9 g		
monounsaturated 1.5 g			

PER SERVING
BLUEBERRY PANCAKES

calories 196	**cholesterol** 1 mg	**protein** 7 g	**dietary exchanges**
total fat 2.5 g	**sodium** 255 mg	**calcium** 199 mg	2½ starch
saturated 0.5 g	**carbohydrates** 36 g	**potassium** 153 mg	
trans 0.0 g	fiber 1 g		
polyunsaturated 1.0 g	sugars 11 g		
monounsaturated 1.5 g			

OATMEAL-BANANA WAFFLES
with Strawberry Sauce

With this recipe in your repertoire, you'll be tempted to start a weekend tradition of serving waffles for a special breakfast treat. Double the recipe when you have guests or so you'll have waffles to freeze for quick breakfasts later on.

SERVES 6 | 1 waffle and 2 tablespoons sauce per serving

In a food processor or blender, process the strawberries and honey until smooth. Pour into a small bowl. Cover and refrigerate until ready to use. (The sauce will keep for up to three days. If you prepare the sauce ahead of time, you may want to let it come to room temperature before spooning it over the waffles.)

In a medium bowl, stir together the buttermilk, oatmeal, banana, egg substitute, brown sugar, and oil until the oatmeal is moistened. Let the mixture stand for 5 minutes to soften the oatmeal.

Meanwhile, preheat a waffle iron using the manufacturer's directions. Preheat the oven to 200°F. Line a baking sheet with aluminum foil. Set aside.

In a small bowl, stir together the flours, baking powder, and baking soda. Whisk into the buttermilk mixture until the batter is just moistened but no flour is visible. Don't overmix; the batter should be slightly lumpy.

SAUCE
- 8 ounces strawberries, hulled and halved
- 1½ teaspoons honey

WAFFLES
- ¾ cup low-fat buttermilk
- ¼ cup uncooked quick-cooking oatmeal
- ½ large banana, mashed
- ¼ cup egg substitute or 2 large eggs
- 1½ tablespoons light brown sugar
- 1½ teaspoons canola or corn oil
- ½ cup all-purpose flour
- ¼ cup whole-wheat flour
- 1 teaspoon baking powder
- ⅛ teaspoon baking soda

Cooking spray
- 2 tablespoons chopped pecans, dry-roasted

Lightly spray the heated waffle iron with cooking spray. Spoon the batter for the first waffle over the waffle iron. Following the manufacturer's directions for timing, cook until the steaming stops and the waffle is golden brown. Watch the first batch closely and adjust the time as necessary. Transfer the waffle to the baking sheet. Put in the oven to keep warm, uncovered, for up to 45 minutes. Repeat with the remaining batter.

Top each waffle with about 2 tablespoons strawberry sauce. Sprinkle each with about 1 teaspoon pecans.

PER SERVING

calories 145
total fat 3.0 g
  saturated 0.5 g
  trans 0.0 g
  polyunsaturated 1.0 g
  monounsaturated 1.5 g

cholesterol 1 mg
sodium 148 mg
carbohydrates 26 g
  fiber 3 g
  sugars 10 g

protein 5 g
calcium 95 mg
potassium 217 mg

dietary exchanges
1½ starch

OVERNIGHT "APPLE PIE" OATMEAL

Assemble the ingredients for this oatmeal in the slow cooker before you go to sleep, and a heart-healthy breakfast reminiscent of apple pie will await you in the morning. Unless you have a large family, you'll even have enough left over for another breakfast later in the week.

SERVES 8 | 1 cup per serving

Heavily spray a 3½- or 4-quart slow cooker with cooking spray. Put the remaining ingredients in the slow cooker, stirring well. Cook, covered, on low for 6 to 7 hours.

Stir the cooked oatmeal before serving.

Don't leave any remaining oatmeal in the slow cooker; it may stick. Spoon it into an airtight container and refrigerate.

To reheat an individual serving, spoon 1 cup of the oatmeal into a microwaveable container and microwave, covered, on 100 percent power (high) for 1 to 2 minutes, or until heated through, stirring once halfway through and adding 1 to 2 tablespoons fat-free milk as necessary for the desired consistency (the oatmeal will have thickened while it was refrigerated).

Cooking spray
- 2 cups uncooked steel-cut oats
- 1 very large unpeeled apple or pear (9 to 10 ounces, any variety), chopped
- ¾ cup sweetened dried cranberries
- ½ cup firmly packed light brown sugar
- 5 cups fat-free milk
- 1 cup water
- 2 teaspoons apple pie spice
- ½ teaspoon vanilla extract

COOK'S TIP ON COOKING OATMEAL IN SLOW COOKERS Steel-cut oats are the best choice for oatmeal prepared in a slow cooker because they can withstand the longer cooking time without getting mushy.

COOK'S TIP ON APPLE PIE SPICE If you don't have apple pie spice on hand but do have pumpkin pie spice, that also will work well here. If you want to make your own blend, it can be as basic as combining equal amounts of ground cinnamon and ground nutmeg. For a mixture more similar to apple pie spice, though, try using four parts of ground cinnamon, two parts each of ground nutmeg and ground cloves, and one part each of ground allspice and ground cardamom. Feel free to adjust the amounts to taste.

PER SERVING

calories 318	**cholesterol** 3 mg	**protein** 11 g	**dietary exchanges**
total fat 3.0 g	**sodium** 70 mg	**calcium** 228 mg	2 starch
saturated 0.0 g	**carbohydrates** 62 g	**potassium** 425 mg	1 fruit
trans 0.0 g	fiber 9 g		1 fat-free milk
polyunsaturated 1.0 g	sugars 33 g		
monounsaturated 1.0 g			

PARADISE SMOOTHIES

A combination of mango, cantaloupe, and banana creates a taste of paradise with just the swirling of the blender.

SERVES 4 | 1 cup per serving

In a small bowl, stir together the wheat germ and cinnamon. Set aside.

In a blender, process the remaining ingredients until smooth. Pour into glasses or wine goblets. Sprinkle with the wheat germ mixture. Serve immediately.

- 1 tablespoon toasted wheat germ
- ¼ teaspoon ground cinnamon
- 8 ounces frozen mango pieces
- 1 cup cantaloupe chunks
- ½ medium banana, cut into 1-inch slices
- 1 cup fresh orange juice
- 1 cup fat-free vanilla yogurt
- ¼ teaspoon vanilla extract

COOK'S TIP ON TOASTED WHEAT GERM

Toasted wheat germ is a nutritious addition to sprinkle on fruit, cereal, or fat-free yogurt or to use as a coating for chicken or fish.

PER SERVING

calories 155	**cholesterol** 1 mg	**protein** 5 g	**dietary exchanges**
total fat 0.5 g	**sodium** 50 mg	**calcium** 128 mg	1½ fruit
saturated 0.0 g	**carbohydrates** 35 g	**potassium** 530 mg	1 fat-free milk
trans 0.0 g	fiber 2 g		
polyunsaturated 0.0 g	sugars 29 g		
monounsaturated 0.0 g			

DESSERTS

CHOCOLATE CAKE

A wonderfully moist cake (partly because of baby-food prunes), it's perfect all on its own—no icing required!

SERVES 24 | 1 slice per serving

Preheat the oven to 375°F. Lightly spray a 13 x 9 x 2-inch cake pan or two 8- or 9-inch square cake pans with cooking spray. Line the pan(s) with wax paper or cooking parchment. Set aside.

In a large bowl, sift together the flour, cocoa powder, and baking powder. Make a well in the center.

In a small bowl, whisk together the water, milk, prunes, oil, and vanilla. Pour into the well in the flour mixture, stirring until well combined. The batter will resemble a thick paste.

In a medium mixing bowl, using an electric mixer on medium-low speed, beat the egg whites until foamy. Add the cream of tartar. Increase the speed to medium. Gradually add the sugar, beating after each addition and gradually increasing the speed until the egg whites form soft peaks. Don't overbeat. Gently fold the egg whites into the batter. Pour into the prepared pan(s), gently smoothing the top(s).

Cooking spray

2½ cups all-purpose flour

⅓ cup unsweetened cocoa powder (dark preferred)

1 tablespoon plus ½ teaspoon baking powder

¾ cup water

⅔ cup fat-free milk

1 4-ounce jar pureed baby-food prunes

¼ cup canola or corn oil

1 teaspoon vanilla extract

4 large egg whites

¼ teaspoon cream of tartar

1¾ cups sugar

Bake for 35 to 40 minutes, or until a wooden toothpick inserted in the center comes out clean. Let cool on a cooling rack for 5 minutes. Turn out onto the cooling rack. Peel off the wax paper or cooking parchment. Serve the cake warm or at room temperature.

COOK'S TIP ON COCOA POWDER Made from roasted cocoa beans with most of the fat (cocoa butter) removed, unsweetened cocoa powder can substitute for solid chocolate in baking recipes. Use 3 tablespoons of cocoa powder plus 1 tablespoon of oil, such as canola or corn, for 1 ounce of unsweetened baking chocolate. You'll cut the total fat by 50 to 75 percent. Cocoa powder has many other advantages. It costs less per ounce than baking chocolate and goes almost twice as far. It blends more easily than baking chocolate, reducing the chance of lumpy batters. If you store cocoa powder in a cool, dry place, it will keep almost indefinitely.

PER SERVING

calories 140	**cholesterol** 0 mg	**protein** 3 g	**dietary exchanges**
total fat 2.5 g	**sodium** 71 mg	**calcium** 47 mg	2 other carbohydrate
saturated 0.0 g	**carbohydrates** 27 g	**potassium** 114 mg	½ fat
trans 0.0 g	fiber 1 g		
polyunsaturated 0.5 g	sugars 16 g		
monounsaturated 1.5 g			

CARROT CAKE

This hefty snack cake gives you a double dose of carrots—such a scrumptious way to eat your vegetables!

SERVES 16 | 2 x 3-inch piece per serving

Preheat the oven to 350°F. Lightly spray a 13 x 9 x 2-inch baking pan with cooking spray. Set aside.

In a medium bowl, stir together the honey and oil until smooth. Stir in the baby-food carrots, egg substitute, and vanilla. Stir in the shredded carrots.

In a large bowl, stir together the remaining cake ingredients. Stir in the carrot mixture. Pour into the baking pan, gently smoothing the top.

Bake for 25 minutes, or until a wooden toothpick inserted in the center comes out clean. Let cool on a cooling rack before slicing.

In a small bowl, stir together the topping ingredients. Top each slice of cake with a dollop of the mixture.

Cooking spray

CAKE
- 1 cup honey
- 2 tablespoons canola or corn oil
- 1 4-ounce jar pureed baby-food carrots
- ¼ cup egg substitute or 2 large egg whites
- 1 teaspoon vanilla extract
- 2 cups shredded carrots
- 1 cup all-purpose flour
- 1 cup whole-wheat flour
- ¼ cup fat-free dry milk
- 2 teaspoons baking powder
- 1 teaspoon ground cinnamon
- ⅛ teaspoon ground nutmeg

TOPPING (optional)
- 2 cups frozen fat-free whipped topping, thawed in refrigerator
- ½ teaspoon ground nutmeg or cinnamon

PER SERVING

calories 148	**cholesterol** 0 mg	**protein** 3 g	**dietary exchanges**
total fat 2.0 g	**sodium** 77 mg	**calcium** 57 mg	2 other carbohydrate
saturated 0.0 g	**carbohydrates** 31 g	**potassium** 135 mg	½ fat
trans 0.0 g	fiber 2 g		
polyunsaturated 0.5 g	sugars 19 g		
monounsaturated 1.0 g			

GINGERBREAD

Adding fresh apple gives this gingerbread a deep sweetness.

SERVES 10 | 1 square per serving

In a medium mixing bowl, stir together the milk and vinegar. Let stand for 10 minutes.

Preheat the oven to 350°F. Lightly spray a 9-inch square baking pan with cooking spray. Set aside.

Meanwhile, in a medium bowl, stir together the flours, ginger, baking soda, and cinnamon. Set aside.

Add the remaining ingredients except the apple to the milk mixture. Using an electric mixer on medium speed, beat until blended.

Gradually add the flour mixture, stirring well after each addition. Fold in the apple. Pour into the pan, gently smoothing the top.

Bake for 30 minutes, or until a wooden toothpick inserted in the center comes out clean. Let cool on a cooling rack for at least 10 minutes before slicing.

1 5-ounce can fat-free evaporated milk

2 teaspoons cider vinegar

Cooking spray

1 cup all-purpose flour

1 cup whole-wheat flour

1 teaspoon ground ginger

½ teaspoon baking soda

½ teaspoon ground cinnamon

¾ cup honey

1 6-ounce jar pureed baby-food sweet potatoes

2 tablespoons egg substitute or 1 large egg white

1 tablespoon plus 2 teaspoons canola or corn oil

½ cup chopped peeled apple

PER SERVING

calories 211
total fat 3.0 g
   saturated 0.5 g
   trans 0.0 g
   polyunsaturated 1.0 g
   monounsaturated 1.5 g

cholesterol 1 mg
sodium 90 mg
carbohydrates 44 g
   fiber 2 g
   sugars 25 g

protein 5 g
calcium 54 mg
potassium 180 mg

dietary exchanges
   3 other carbohydrate
   ½ fat

GINGERBREAD COOKIE CUTOUTS

You'll know the holidays have arrived when the spicy aroma of gingerbread cookies fills your home!

SERVES 18 | 2 4-inch cookies per serving

In a large bowl, stir together the brown sugar, molasses, oil, egg substitute, and sugar.

In a medium bowl, stir together 3 cups flour, the baking powder, cinnamon, ginger, baking soda, cloves, and salt. Gradually add to the brown sugar mixture, stirring to form a soft dough. Return the dough to the medium bowl, cover tightly, and refrigerate for 2 to 12 hours.

Preheat the oven to 375°F. Lightly spray two baking sheets with cooking spray. Set aside.

Sprinkle the remaining flour on a flat work surface. Roll half the cookie dough to ⅛-inch thickness. Dip the edges of cookie cutters in flour, shaking off the excess. Cut out the cookies, continuing to dip the cookie cutters in flour as needed to keep the dough from sticking. Transfer the cookies to one of the baking sheets. Repeat with the remaining dough.

¾ cup firmly packed light brown sugar

½ cup molasses (dark preferred)

¼ cup canola or corn oil

¼ cup egg substitute or 1 large egg

2 tablespoons sugar

3 cups all-purpose flour (plus more as needed for making dough)

1 teaspoon baking powder

1 teaspoon ground cinnamon

1 teaspoon ground ginger

½ teaspoon baking soda

½ teaspoon ground cloves

¼ teaspoon salt

Cooking spray

Bake for 5 to 6 minutes, or until the cookies are slightly firm to the touch (they shouldn't brown). Transfer the baking sheets to cooling racks. Let the cookies cool slightly. Transfer the cookies to the cooling racks. When the cookies have cooled completely, store them in airtight tins for up to one week.

COOK'S TIP ON MOLASSES A by-product of sugar refining, molasses is available in three grades: light (or mild), dark, and blackstrap. Light molasses is the lightest in body and color and the sweetest in taste. Many pancake and waffle syrups include light molasses, which can replace or supplement sugar or honey in some cooking. Dark molasses is more robust, thicker, less sweet, and darker in color. Its distinct flavor spices up foods such as gingerbread, gingerbread cookies, and baked beans. Light and dark molasses are interchangeable, depending on your taste preference; blackstrap molasses, however, is bitter and shouldn't be used unless your recipe specifically calls for it.

PER SERVING

calories 172	**cholesterol** 0 mg	**protein** 3 g	**dietary exchanges**
total fat 3.5 g	**sodium** 103 mg	**calcium** 45 mg	2 other carbohydrate
saturated 0.5 g	**carbohydrates** 33 g	**potassium** 172 mg	½ fat
trans 0.0 g	fiber 1 g		
polyunsaturated 1.0 g	sugars 15 g		
monounsaturated 2.0 g			

PEACH AND BLUEBERRY COBBLER

A rustic whole-wheat biscuit topping complements the lightly sweetened fruit of this homey dessert.

SERVES 8 | ¾ cup fruit mixture and 1 "biscuit" per serving

Preheat the oven to 425°F. Lightly spray an 11 x 7 x 2-inch glass baking dish with cooking spray. Set aside.

In a large bowl, combine the filling ingredients, gently stirring with a rubber scraper. Spoon into the baking dish.

Bake for 20 minutes, or until the filling is bubbly at the edges. Transfer the baking dish to a cooling rack. (Leave the oven on.)

Meanwhile, in a medium bowl, stir together the whole-wheat flour, remaining ¼ cup all-purpose flour, ¼ cup sugar, the baking powder, and baking soda. Pour in the buttermilk and oil, stirring until the dough is just moistened but no flour is visible.

Cooking spray

FILLING

- 3 **pounds fresh peaches, peeled and sliced, or 2 pounds frozen unsweetened sliced peaches, thawed if frozen**
- 1 **cup fresh or frozen blueberries (don't thaw if frozen)**
- 2 **tablespoons sugar**
- 2 **tablespoons all-purpose flour**
- 1 **teaspoon grated lemon zest**
- ½ **teaspoon ground cinnamon**

TOPPING

- ½ **cup whole-wheat flour**
- ¼ **cup all-purpose flour**
- ¼ **cup sugar and 1 tablespoon sugar, divided use**
- ½ **teaspoon baking powder**

(continued)

When the filling is ready, using scant ¼ cup measures to make 8 mounds of dough, spoon the topping onto the filling. Sprinkle the cobbler with the remaining 1 tablespoon sugar.

Bake for 15 minutes, or until the topping is puffed and lightly browned. Transfer to a cooling rack and let cool for 15 to 20 minutes. Serve warm.

¼ teaspoon baking soda
½ cup low-fat buttermilk
2 tablespoons canola or corn oil

COOK'S TIP ON CITRUS ZEST An implement called a zester makes quick work of removing the peel, or zest, of citrus fruit. Use rather firm downward strokes, being careful to avoid cutting into any of the pith, the white bitter covering just beneath the peel. Measuring will be easy if you work over a small plate.

PER SERVING

calories 195	**cholesterol** 1 mg	**protein** 4 g	**dietary exchanges**
total fat 4.5 g	**sodium** 81 mg	**calcium** 48 mg	1 starch
saturated 0.5 g	**carbohydrates** 39 g	**potassium** 357 mg	1 fruit
trans 0.0 g	fiber 4 g		½ other carbohydrate
polyunsaturated 1.0 g	sugars 26 g		½ fat
monounsaturated 2.5 g			

NECTARINE CRUMBLE

Sliced almonds add crunch to the crumbles topping plump slices of sweet, firm-fleshed nectarines in this fragrant dessert.

SERVES 8 | ½ cup per serving

Preheat the oven to 375°F.

In a medium bowl, stir together the nectarines, ¼ cup brown sugar, the orange juice concentrate, lemon zest, almond extract, and nutmeg. Pour into an 8-inch square nonstick baking pan. Set aside.

In a small bowl, using a fork, stir together the oatmeal, almonds, flour, margarine, cinnamon, and remaining 1 tablespoon brown sugar until the margarine is distributed throughout. Sprinkle over the nectarine mixture.

Bake for 30 to 35 minutes, or until the nectarines are tender and the topping is golden brown.

2 pounds fresh unpeeled nectarines, sliced, or 2½ pounds frozen unsweetened sliced peaches, thawed

¼ cup firmly packed light brown sugar and 1 tablespoon firmly packed light brown sugar, divided use

2 tablespoons frozen orange juice concentrate

1 teaspoon grated lemon zest

½ teaspoon almond extract

¼ teaspoon ground nutmeg

½ cup uncooked quick-cooking oatmeal

3 tablespoons sliced almonds

2 tablespoons all-purpose flour

1 tablespoon light tub margarine

½ teaspoon ground cinnamon

PER SERVING

calories 131	**cholesterol** 0 mg	**protein** 3 g	**dietary exchanges**
total fat 2.5 g	**sodium** 14 mg	**calcium** 26 mg	2 other carbohydrate
saturated 0.0 g	**carbohydrates** 27 g	**potassium** 286 mg	½ fat
trans 0.0 g	fiber 3 g		
polyunsaturated 0.5 g	sugars 18 g		
monounsaturated 1.0 g			

FLAN CARAMEL

Spoon sliced peaches or nectarines and caramel topping over these extra-creamy flans for a special treat.

SERVES 6 | ½ cup per serving

Preheat the oven to 325°F. Lightly spray six 6-ounce custard cups with cooking spray.

In a large bowl, whisk together the milk, egg, egg whites, sugar, sherry, vanilla, and nutmeg. Pour about ½ cup of the mixture into each custard cup. Place the custard cups in a large pan with a rim. Place the pan in the oven and carefully pour hot water into the large pan to a depth of about 1 inch. Be sure the water doesn't get into the custard cups.

Bake for 50 minutes, or until a wooden toothpick or knife inserted near the center of a flan comes out clean. Remove the custard cups from the pan and let cool completely on a cooling rack. Cover and refrigerate until serving time (up to 24 hours). Run a knife around the edge of a flan, place a dessert plate on top, and invert to remove the flan. Repeat with the remaining flans.

Just before serving the flans, in a small microwaveable bowl, microwave the caramel topping on 100 percent power (high) for 10 seconds. Spoon the topping and peaches over each serving. Serve immediately.

Cooking spray
2½ cups fat-free milk
1 large egg
2 large egg whites
¼ cup sugar
1 tablespoon dry or sweet sherry
1 teaspoon vanilla extract
Dash of ground nutmeg
¼ cup plus 2 tablespoons fat-free caramel ice cream topping
1½ cups sliced peeled peaches or sliced nectarines

PER SERVING

calories 168	**cholesterol** 37 mg	**protein** 6 g	**dietary exchanges**
total fat 1.0 g	**sodium** 128 mg	**calcium** 132 mg	½ fat-free milk
saturated 0.5 g	**carbohydrates** 33 g	**potassium** 265 mg	1½ other carbohydrate
trans 0.0 g	fiber 1 g		
polyunsaturated 0.0 g	sugars 27 g		
monounsaturated 0.5 g			

BERRY NAPOLEONS

When berries are at their peak, use them to make a gorgeous dessert fit for an emperor—or your family! The crisp wonton wrappers are a low-fat stand-in for the puff pastry typically used to make napoleons.

SERVES 4 | 1 napoleon per serving

Preheat the oven to 375°F.

Place the wonton wrappers in a single layer on a large baking pan. Brush both sides of each wrapper with the oil.

Bake for 8 to 10 minutes, or until golden brown. Transfer the pan to a cooling rack and let the wrappers cool for about 10 minutes.

Meanwhile, put the thawed raspberries in a fine-mesh sieve over a medium bowl. Using a rubber scraper, press the berries through the sieve. Discard the solids. Add the sugar to the raspberry sauce, stirring until the sugar is dissolved. Set aside.

Place 1 wonton wrapper on each plate. Sprinkle half the strawberries and half the blueberries over the wonton wrappers. Drizzle each serving with 2 teaspoons raspberry sauce. Repeat with another layer of wonton wrappers and the remaining strawberries and blueberries. Drizzle each serving with 2 teaspoons raspberry

12 wonton wrappers

2 teaspoons canola or corn oil

10 ounces frozen unsweetened raspberries, thawed

1 tablespoon sugar

⅔ cup sliced strawberries

⅔ cup blueberries

⅔ cup raspberries

¼ teaspoon confectioners' sugar

sauce. Top each with another wonton wrapper. Drizzle the plates with the remaining raspberry sauce. Sprinkle the fresh raspberries over the sauce. Sprinkle the tops of the napoleons with the confectioners' sugar.

COOK'S TIP You can bake the wonton wrappers a day ahead and store them at room temperature in an airtight container. Assemble the napoleons just before serving.

PER SERVING

calories 183	**cholesterol** 2 mg	**protein** 4 g	**dietary exchanges**
total fat 3.0 g	**sodium** 16 mg	**calcium** 40 mg	1 starch
saturated 0.5 g	**carbohydrates** 37 g	**potassium** 220 mg	1½ fruit
trans 0.0 g	fiber 6 g		½ fat
polyunsaturated 1.0 g	sugars 13 g		
monounsaturated 1.5 g			

LEMON CREAM
with Raspberries and Gingersnap Topping

Terrific all by itself, this lemon cream is even more delicious with a double dose of raspberries, plus gingersnaps and lemon zest.

SERVES 6 | ½ cup per serving

In a small bowl, stir together the gingersnap crumbs and lemon zest. Sprinkle a thin layer into dessert bowls or wine goblets. Set the remaining mixture aside.

Put the boiling water and gelatin in a food processor or blender. Process until the gelatin is dissolved.

If using ice cubes, stir them into the gelatin mixture until well blended or the ice has melted. If using cold water, stir until well blended.

Add the whipped topping and cream cheese and process until smooth. Pour into the dessert bowls or wine goblets. Refrigerate until firm, about 1 hour.

Meanwhile, in another small bowl, gently stir together 1½ cups raspberries and the confectioners' sugar and vanilla. Pour into a fine-mesh sieve. Using a rubber scraper, press the mixture back into the bowl. Discard the solids. Set aside.

When the gelatin is firm, top with the raspberry mixture, then with the remaining gingersnap mixture. Garnish with the remaining ¼ cup plus 2 tablespoons raspberries.

8 low-fat gingersnaps (lowest sodium available), finely crushed

1 teaspoon grated lemon zest

¾ cup boiling water

1 box (4-serving size) sugar-free lemon gelatin

1 cup ice cubes or ⅔ cup cold water

1 cup frozen fat-free whipped topping, thawed in refrigerator

2 ounces fat-free cream cheese

1½ cups fresh or frozen unsweetened raspberries, thawed if frozen, and ¼ cup plus 2 tablespoons fresh raspberries (optional), divided use

1 tablespoon confectioners' sugar

¼ teaspoon vanilla extract

COOK'S TIP ON STORING FRESH RASPBERRIES Fresh raspberries are quite perishable, so don't count on keeping them in the refrigerator for more than a day or two after you buy them. Remove them from the container as soon as you get them home, and discard any moldy berries to keep the mold from spreading to the other berries. Blot the remaining berries with paper towels. If you aren't going to eat the berries the day of purchase, spread the unrinsed berries in a shallow pan or on a plate, cover them with paper towels, then wrap the pan or plate in plastic wrap. For longer storage, first rinse the berries, drain them thoroughly, and pat them dry with paper towels. Spread them in a single layer on a baking sheet with shallow sides and freeze them. When they are solidly frozen, transfer them to an airtight plastic freezer bag and keep frozen for up to nine months.

COOK'S TIP ON USING FROZEN RASPBERRIES You don't need to thaw frozen raspberries before using them in recipes, but you may need to add a few minutes to the cooking time. Also, frozen berries exude more juice than their fresh counterparts, so when using frozen berries in pies, cobblers, crisps, and similar dishes, use less liquid and more thickener.

PER SERVING

calories 93	**cholesterol** 2 mg	**protein** 3 g	**dietary exchanges**
total fat 1.0 g	**sodium** 150 mg	**calcium** 61 mg	1 other carbohydrate
saturated 0.5 g	**carbohydrates** 16 g	**potassium** 68 mg	
trans 0.0 g	fiber 2 g		
polyunsaturated 0.0 g	sugars 7 g		
monounsaturated 0.5 g			

RICE PUDDING
with Caramelized Bananas

Bananas are a good source of potassium, which is an important nutrient for lowering blood pressure. These bananas, enhanced with brown sugar, cinnamon, and vanilla extract, crown brown rice pudding, which is served barely warm.

SERVES 6 | ½ cup rice pudding and scant ¼ cup banana per serving

In a medium saucepan, bring the water to a boil over high heat. Add the rice. Reduce the heat and simmer, uncovered, for 30 minutes. Drain well in a colander.

Preheat the oven to 350°F. Lightly spray a 1-quart glass baking dish with cooking spray.

In a medium bowl, stir together the rice, milk, egg substitute, sugar, 2 teaspoons vanilla, ½ teaspoon cinnamon, and the nutmeg. Pour into the baking dish. Cover the dish and set it in a large baking pan. Pour hot tap water into the pan to a depth of 1 inch.

Bake for 1 hour, or until the mixture thickens. Remove from the oven and let stand for 20 to 30 minutes, or until barely warm.

Near the end of the standing time, melt the margarine in a medium nonstick skillet over medium-high heat, swirling to coat the bottom. Add the bananas, brown sugar, and remaining ¼ teaspoon cinnamon, stirring gently to coat.

10 cups water

½ cup plus 2 tablespoons uncooked brown rice

Cooking spray

2 cups fat-free milk

½ cup egg substitute

¼ cup sugar

2 teaspoons vanilla extract and ¼ teaspoon vanilla extract, divided use

½ teaspoon ground cinnamon and ¼ teaspoon ground cinnamon, divided use

¼ teaspoon ground nutmeg (level or heaping)

2 tablespoons light tub margarine

2 medium bananas, cut crosswise into ⅜-inch slices

1 tablespoon firmly packed dark brown sugar

Cook for 1 to 2 minutes, or until the bananas are soft and glossy, stirring constantly and gently. Remove from the heat. Gently stir in the remaining ¼ teaspoon vanilla.

Spoon the pudding into bowls. Spoon the bananas over the pudding.

SPICED FRUIT

You will need to make this colorful dessert at least 8 hours in advance. If you want to stretch it to serve 12, spoon a half-cup of fat-free vanilla frozen yogurt into each bowl and top each serving with a half-cup of Spiced Fruit.

SERVES 8 | ¾ cup per serving

In a medium saucepan, stir together the brown sugar, sauterne, vinegar, cloves, and curry powder. Add the cinnamon sticks. Cook over medium heat for 3 to 5 minutes, or until heated through, stirring frequently.

Meanwhile, in a large bowl, stir together the remaining ingredients.

Pour the hot syrup over the fruit. Stir well. Let cool at room temperature for 30 minutes. Cover and refrigerate for 8 to 24 hours. Discard the cloves and cinnamon sticks before serving the fruit.

1 cup firmly packed light brown sugar

½ cup sauterne, dry white wine (regular or nonalcoholic), or apple juice

¼ cup cider vinegar

10 to 15 whole cloves

⅛ teaspoon curry powder

2 cinnamon sticks, each about 3 inches long

1 15-ounce can sliced peaches in fruit juice, drained

1 15-ounce can sliced pears in fruit juice, drained

16 to 24 honeydew melon balls, fresh or frozen, or 4 medium kiwifruit, peeled and sliced

8 fresh pineapple spears or one 20-ounce can pineapple chunks in their own juice, drained

2 to 4 plums, sliced

PER SERVING

calories 222
total fat 0.0 g
  saturated 0.0 g
  trans 0.0 g
  polyunsaturated 0.0 g
  monounsaturated 0.0 g

cholesterol 0 mg
sodium 25 mg
carbohydrates 54 g
  fiber 2 g
  sugars 48 g

protein 1 g
calcium 36 mg
potassium 290 mg

dietary exchanges
  1½ fruit
  2 other carbohydrate

MANGO AND PAPAYA

with Ricotta Cream

Easy enough for weeknights and special enough for guests, this dessert pairs cool and creamy ricotta cheese with liqueur-soaked fruits. You can substitute two cups of almost any other fruit you like, and you may want to try other flavors of liqueur as well.

SERVES 4 | ½ cup fruit and 2 tablespoons ricotta cream per serving

In a medium bowl, stir together the mango, papaya, and liqueur. Let stand at room temperature for 30 minutes, stirring occasionally.

Meanwhile, in a food processor or blender, process the ricotta and sugar until smooth. Transfer to a small bowl. Stir in the lime zest. Cover and refrigerate until the mango mixture has macerated.

To serve, spoon the mango mixture into shallow dishes. Drizzle each serving with the ricotta cream. Sprinkle each with coconut.

½ medium mango, sliced

½ small papaya, seeded and sliced

1 tablespoon orange liqueur or fresh orange juice

½ cup fat-free ricotta cheese

1 tablespoon sugar

¼ teaspoon grated lime zest

2 tablespoons sweetened flaked coconut, toasted

PER SERVING

calories 84	**cholesterol** 3 mg	**protein** 4 g	**dietary exchanges**
total fat 1.0 g	**sodium** 69 mg	**calcium** 133 mg	1 other carbohydrate
saturated 0.5 g	**carbohydrates** 13 g	**potassium** 142 mg	½ very lean meat
trans 0.0 g	fiber 1 g		
polyunsaturated 0.0 g	sugars 12 g		
monounsaturated 0.0 g			

ICE CREAM
with Hot Tropical Fruit

Bananas Foster goes tropical with the addition of pineapple and toasted coconut.

SERVES 4 | ½ cup ice cream and ¼ cup banana mixture per serving

In a large nonstick skillet, melt the margarine over medium-high heat, swirling to coat the bottom. Gently stir in the bananas, pineapple, brown sugar, and cinnamon. Cook for 2 minutes, or until the bananas are soft and glossy, stirring gently and constantly. Remove from the heat. Stir in the vanilla.

Just before serving, spoon the ice cream into dessert bowls. Spoon the banana mixture over each serving. Sprinkle with the coconut. Serve immediately.

COOK'S TIP ON TOASTING COCONUT Heat a nonstick skillet over medium-high heat. Toast the coconut for 1 to 2 minutes, or until it begins to brown on the edges, stirring constantly. Transfer to a plate to stop the toasting.

2 tablespoons light tub margarine

2 medium bananas, sliced

4 ounces canned pineapple chunks, packed in their own juice, drained and halved

2 tablespoons firmly packed light or dark brown sugar

½ teaspoon ground cinnamon

½ teaspoon vanilla extract

2 cups fat-free vanilla ice cream or frozen yogurt

2 tablespoons sweetened flaked coconut, toasted

PER SERVING

calories 224	**cholesterol** 0 mg	**protein** 4 g	**dietary exchanges**
total fat 3.0 g	**sodium** 121 mg	**calcium** 118 mg	1 fruit
saturated 1.0 g	**carbohydrates** 47 g	**potassium** 476 mg	2 other carbohydrate
trans 0.0 g	fiber 3 g		½ fat
polyunsaturated 0.5 g	sugars 23 g		
monounsaturated 1.5 g			

STRAWBERRY-BANANA SORBET

When the bananas on your counter start to freckle, it's time to make sorbet!

SERVES 6 | ½ cup per serving

Put the strawberries and bananas in a large airtight plastic bag. Place the bag in the freezer so the fruit is in a single layer. Freeze for 2 to 3 hours, or until firm (the fruit will still be very slightly soft).

In a food processor or blender, process all the ingredients except the kiwifruit until smooth. Stir in the kiwifruit. Serve the sorbet immediately (it will be slightly soft), or return it to the freezer for 1 to 2 hours, or until it reaches the desired texture. If you freeze the sorbet (up to one month), remove it from the freezer 5 to 10 minutes before serving to soften slightly.

1 pound fresh strawberries, hulled and halved, or 1 pound frozen unsweetened strawberries, slightly thawed

2 large bananas, cut into ½-inch slices

¼ cup firmly packed light brown sugar

2 tablespoons pineapple juice

1 teaspoon grated lemon zest

2 medium kiwifruit, peeled, sliced, and mashed with a fork

COOK'S TIP ON KIWIFRUIT When kiwifruit seeds are chopped in a food processor or blender, they impart a bitter flavor. That is why it is best to mash kiwifruit with a fork.

PER SERVING

calories 118	**cholesterol** 0 mg	**protein** 1 g	**dietary exchanges**
total fat 0.5 g	**sodium** 5 mg	**calcium** 31 mg	2 fruit
saturated 0.0 g	**carbohydrates** 30 g	**potassium** 376 mg	
trans 0.0 g	fiber 4 g		
polyunsaturated 0.0 g	sugars 21 g		
monounsaturated 0.0 g			

FROZEN MINI CHOCOLATE MOUSSE SOUFFLÉS

Fear of falling? Not with these frosty, airy soufflés.

SERVES 8 | ½ cup per serving

In a medium bowl, whisk together the milk, cocoa powder, and vanilla until the cocoa powder is incorporated. Set aside.

In a large mixing bowl, whisk together the water and powdered egg whites. Let stand for 2 to 3 minutes, or until the egg whites are rehydrated. Using an electric mixer on medium-low speed, beat until foamy. Increase the speed to medium high and continue beating until the mixture forms stiff peaks.

Pour the milk mixture over the egg whites. Fold in with a rubber scraper.

Fold in the whipped topping. Ladle the mixture into eight 6-ounce glass or ceramic custard cups. Cover the custard cups and place on a tray if desired. Freeze for 4 hours, or until the soufflés are firm. The soufflés will keep in the freezer for up to one month.

1 14-ounce can fat-free sweetened condensed milk

¼ cup unsweetened cocoa powder (dark preferred)

1 teaspoon vanilla extract

½ cup warm water

2 tablespoons plus 2 teaspoons powdered egg whites (pasteurized dried egg whites)

1 cup frozen fat-free whipped topping, thawed in refrigerator

PER SERVING

calories 176
total fat 0.5 g
  saturated 0.0 g
  trans 0.0 g
  polyunsaturated 0.0 g
  monounsaturated 0.0 g

cholesterol 3 mg
sodium 85 mg
carbohydrates 35 g
  fiber 1 g
  sugars 32 g

protein 6 g
calcium 129 mg
potassium 346 mg

dietary exchanges
  ½ fat-free milk
  2 other carbohydrate

RESOURCES

MY SODIUM TRACKER

DATE: _____ ☐ Mon ☐ Tues ☐ Wed ☐ Thurs ☐ Fri ☐ Sat ☐ Sun

TIME/PLACE	FOOD OR BEVERAGE (TYPE AND AMOUNT)	SODIUM (MG)
BREAKFAST		
SNACK		
LUNCH		
SNACK		
DINNER		
SNACK		
	DAILY TOTAL:	

NOTES

NO-SODIUM SEASONING GUIDE

Try these suggested seasonings to add flavor instead of salt to your at-home cooking.

BREADS	Anise, caraway seeds, cardamom, fennel, poppy seeds, sesame seeds
DESSERTS	Anise, caraway seeds, cardamom, cinnamon, cloves, coriander, ginger, mace, mint, nutmeg, poppy seeds
ENTRÉES	
Beef	Allspice, bay leaf, bell pepper, cayenne, cumin, curry powder, garlic, marjoram, mushrooms, dry mustard, nutmeg, onion, rosemary, sage, thyme, wine
Pork	Apple, applesauce, cinnamon, cloves, fennel, garlic, ginger, mint, onion, sage, savory, wine
Poultry	Basil, bay leaf, bell pepper, cinnamon, curry powder, garlic, lemon juice, marjoram, mushrooms, onion, paprika, parsley, lemon pepper, rosemary, saffron, sage, savory, sesame, tarragon, thyme, wine
Seafood	Allspice, basil, bay leaf, bell pepper, cayenne, cumin, curry powder, fennel, garlic, lemon juice, mace, marjoram, mint, mushrooms, dry mustard, onion, paprika, saffron, sage, sesame seeds, tarragon, thyme, turmeric, wine
SALADS	Basil, chervil, coriander, dill, lemon juice, mint, mustard, oregano, parsley, rosemary, sage, savory, sesame seeds, turmeric, vinegar, watercress
VEGETABLES	
Asparagus	Garlic, lemon juice, onion
Beans, Dried	Caraway seeds, cloves, cumin, mint, savory, tarragon, thyme
Carrots	Anise, cinnamon, cloves, mint, sage, tarragon
Corn	Allspice, bell pepper, cumin, pimiento, tomato
Cucumbers	Chives, dill, garlic, vinegar
Green Beans	Dill, lemon juice, marjoram, nutmeg, pimiento
Greens	Garlic, lemon juice, onion, vinegar
Peas	Allspice, bell pepper, mint, mushrooms, onions, parsley, sage, savory
Potatoes	Bell pepper, chives, dill, garlic, onion, pimiento, saffron
Squash	Allspice, brown sugar, cinnamon, cloves, fennel, ginger, mace, nutmeg, onion
Tomatoes	Allspice, basil, garlic, marjoram, onion, oregano, sage, savory, tarragon, thyme

FOOD GROUPS & SUGGESTED SERVINGS

The following chart lists an average number of recommended servings of each food group based on daily calorie intake. The number of servings that is right for you will vary depending on your caloric needs. Choose foods that are low in sodium, saturated fat, trans fats, and cholesterol and don't have added sugars. When shopping, compare nutrition facts panels and look for the products that are lowest in sodium.

FOOD GROUP	CALORIE RANGE			SAMPLE SERVING SIZES
	1,600	**2,000**	**2,600**	
Vegetables Eat a variety of colors and types.	3 to 4 servings per day	4 to 5 servings per day	5 to 6 servings per day	1 cup raw leafy vegetable ½ cup cut-up raw or cooked nonleafy vegetable ½ cup vegetable juice
Fruits Eat a variety of colors and types.	4 servings per day	4 to 5 servings per day	5 to 6 servings per day	1 medium fruit ¼ cup dried fruit ½ cup fresh, frozen, or canned fruit ½ cup fruit juice
Fiber-rich whole grains Choose whole grains for at least half of your servings.	6 servings per day	6 to 8 servings per day	10 to 11 servings per day	1 slice bread 1 oz dry cereal (check nutrition label for cup measurements) ½ cup cooked rice, pasta, or cereal

FOOD GROUP	CALORIE RANGE			SAMPLE SERVING SIZES
	1,600	2,000	2,600	
Fat-free, 1% fat, and low-fat dairy products Choose fat-free when possible, but compare sodium levels.	2 to 3 servings per day	2 to 3 servings per day	3 servings per day	1 cup milk 1 cup yogurt 1½ oz cheese
Fish Choose varieties rich in omega-3 fatty acids.	6 to 7 oz (cooked) per week	6 to 7 oz (cooked) per week	6 to 7 oz (cooked) per week	3 to 3½ oz cooked fish
Lean meats and skinless poultry Choose lean and extra-lean.	Less than 3 oz (cooked) per day	3 to 6 oz (cooked) per day	6 oz (cooked) per day	3 oz cooked meat or poultry
Legumes, nuts, and seeds Choose unsalted products.	3 servings per week	4 to 5 servings per week	1 serving per day	⅓ cup or 1½ oz nuts 2 Tb peanut butter 2 Tb or ½ oz seeds ½ cup cooked dried beans or peas
Fats and oils Use liquid vegetable oil and spray or light tub margarines most often. Choose products with the lowest amount of sodium.	2 servings per day	2 to 3 servings per day	2 to 3 servings per day	1 tsp light tub margarine 1 Tb light mayonnaise 1 tsp vegetable oil 1 Tb regular or 2 Tb light salad dressing (fat-free dressing does not count as a serving)

Adapted from the DASH eating plan (Dietary Approaches to Stop Hypertension) developed by the National Heart, Lung, and Blood Institute, National Institutes of Health.

COMMON HIGH-SODIUM FOODS

Check this list for an estimate of how much sodium you might find in the commercially prepared versions of some popular high-sodium foods. It's important to be aware of the sources of "hidden" sodium and to look for salt-free or lowest-sodium versions when you buy them. Different manufacturers' products vary greatly, so always read nutrition facts panels and ask for nutrition information at restaurants so you'll know exactly what you're buying.

FOOD OR BEVERAGE	SODIUM (MG)	CALORIES
BREADS AND BREAD PRODUCTS		
English muffin (plain), 2 halves	264	134
Rye, 1 slice	211	83
White, 1 slice	170	66
Whole wheat, 1 slice	132	69
CEREALS (UNCOOKED)		
Bran, ½ cup	75	81
Cornflakes, 1 cup	202	101
Oat circles, 1 cup	186	103
CHEESES		
Brie, 1 ounce	178	95
Cheddar, 1 ounce	176	114
Colby, 1 ounce	171	112
Feta, 1 ounce	316	75
Swiss, 1 ounce	54	108
CONDIMENTS		
Barbecue sauce, ¼ cup	783	105
Chili sauce, 1 tablespoon	230	15
Ketchup, 1 tablespoon	167	15
Mustard, yellow, 1 tablespoon	170	10
Relish, pickle, sweet, 1 tablespoon	124	20

FOOD OR BEVERAGE	SODIUM (MG)	CALORIES
Soy sauce, regular, 1 tablespoon	902	8
Steak sauce, tomato base, 1 tablespoon	227	9
Worcestershire sauce, 1 tablespoon	167	13

MEATS, PROCESSED OR CURED

Bacon, pork, 2 slices	370	87
Bologna, low-fat, 2 slices	626	113
Ham, 96% fat-free, 2 slices	713	60
Hot dog, 96% fat-free beef and pork, 1 hot dog	716	88
Salami, hard, beef and pork, 2 slices	362	69
Sausage, smoked link, beef and pork, 2 links	375	100

SALAD DRESSINGS, REGULAR COMMERCIAL

Blue cheese, 2 tablespoons	279	143
Caesar, 2 tablespoons	317	159
French, 2 tablespoons	268	146
Italian, 2 tablespoons	486	86
Ranch, 2 tablespoons	245	145
Thousand Island, 2 tablespoons	276	118

MISCELLANEOUS

Baking soda, 1 teaspoon	1,259	0
Capers, 1 tablespoon	255	2
Olives, black, 2 large	77	10
Pickles, dill, 1 4-inch pickle	1,181	16
Pizza, chain restaurant, pepperoni, 1 slice of a 14-inch pie	608	324
Vegetable juice, regular, 8 ounces	620	50

We've included some examples for each category, but of course there are many foods we didn't list. Be sure to watch for other foods that also can contain high amounts of sodium, such as:

- Frozen entrées, including pizzas
- Frozen vegetables with sauces
- Canned vegetables
- Canned soups, prepared soup mixes, and bouillon cubes or granules
- Snacks such as crackers, chips, and salted nuts
- Seasonings such as onion salt, garlic salt, monosodium glutamate, and meat tenderizers

GOOD SOURCES OF POTASSIUM

Potassium is considered to be an important component of a dietary approach to lowering blood pressure. Use the list below to add more potassium to your daily diet.

FOOD OR BEVERAGE	POTASSIUM (MG)	SODIUM (MG)	CALORIES
Potato, russet, 1 medium with skin	888	11	168
Yogurt, plain, fat-free, 1 cup	625	189	137
Halibut, Atlantic or Pacific, 3 ounces cooked weight	490	59	119
White beans, canned, no salt added, ½ cup	455	0	110
Tomato sauce, canned, no salt added, ½ cup	453	13	51
Tomatoes, canned, no salt added, 1 cup	451	24	41
Acorn squash, ½ cup cubed	448	4	57
Sweet potato, 1 medium	440	70	100
Cantaloupe, 1 cup cubed	427	26	54
Banana, 1 medium	422	1	105
Spinach, ½ cup cooked	419	63	21
Peaches, dried, ¼ cup	398	3	96
Plums, dried (prunes), ½ cup stewed	398	1	133
Honeydew melon, 1 cup cubed	388	31	61
Milk, fat-free, 1 cup	382	103	83
Apricots, dried, ¼ cup	378	3	78
Trout, rainbow, farm raised, 3 ounces cooked weight	375	36	144
Lima beans, green, ½ cup cooked	365	3	115
Lentils, ½ cup cooked	365	2	115
Kidney beans, ½ cup cooked	358	1	112
Prune juice, ½ cup	353	5	91

FOOD OR BEVERAGE	POTASSIUM (MG)	SODIUM (MG)	CALORIES
Edamame (green soybeans), ½ cup cooked	338	5	95
Top sirloin, fat discarded, 3 ounces cooked weight	334	54	156
Nectarine, 1 large	314	0	69
Pork chop, center loin, 3 ounces cooked weight	303	48	153
Tomato juice, canned, no salt added, ½ cup	278	12	21
Orange juice, ½ cup	248	1	56
Orange, 1 medium	237	0	62
Carrot, raw, 1 large	230	50	30
Plums, dried (prunes), ¼ cup uncooked	220	4	68
Brussels sprouts, fresh, ½ cup cooked	171	11	19

INGREDIENT EQUIVALENTS

Once you've chosen a recipe to prepare, refer to this chart before shopping so you'll know approximately how much to buy of these common ingredients.

INGREDIENT	MEASUREMENT
Almonds	1 ounce = ¼ cup slivers
Apple	1 medium = ¾ to 1 cup chopped; 1 cup sliced
Basil leaves, fresh	⅔ ounce = ½ cup leaves, chopped
Bell pepper, any color	1 medium = 1 cup chopped or sliced
Carrot	1 medium = ⅓ to ½ cup chopped or sliced; ½ cup shredded
Celery	1 medium rib = ½ cup chopped or sliced
Cheese, hard, such as Parmesan	3½ ounces = 1 cup shredded; 4 ounces = 1 cup grated
Cheese, semihard, such as Cheddar, mozzarella, or Swiss	4 ounces = 1 cup grated
Cheese, soft, such as blue, feta, or goat	1 ounce = ¼ cup crumbled
Cucumber	1 medium = 1 cup sliced
Lemon juice	1 medium = 2 to 3 tablespoons
Lemon zest	1 medium = 2 to 3 teaspoons
Lime juice	1 medium = 1½ to 2 tablespoons
Lime zest	1 medium = 1 teaspoon
Mushrooms (button)	1 pound = 5 to 6 cups sliced or chopped
Onions, green	8 to 9 medium = 1 cup sliced (green and white parts)
Onions, white or yellow	1 large = 1 cup chopped; 1 medium = ½ to ⅔ cup chopped; 1 small = ⅓ cup chopped
Orange juice	1 medium = ⅓ to ½ cup
Orange zest	1 medium = 1½ to 2 tablespoons
Strawberries	1 pint = 2 cups sliced or chopped
Tomatoes	2 large, 3 medium, or 4 small = 1½ to 2 cups chopped
Walnuts	1 ounce = ¼ cup chopped

INGREDIENT SUBSTITUTIONS

There's no need to toss out old family recipes and holiday treats because you're watching your sodium intake. Just make a few simple ingredient substitutions to keep enjoying many of your favorite recipes.

IF YOUR RECIPE CALLS FOR	USE
Regular broth or bouillon	Fat-free, salt-free, or very low sodium broths, such as Chicken Broth (page 50), Beef Broth (page 52), Vegetable Broth (page 53), or commercially prepared versions; salt-free or very low sodium bouillon granules or cubes, reconstituted using package directions
Butter or shortening	When possible, use fat-free spray margarine or light tub margarine. Choose the product that is lowest in saturated and trans fats
Butter for sautéing	Vegetable oil, such as canola, corn, or olive; cooking spray; fat-free, low-sodium broth; wine; fruit juice; no-salt-added vegetable juice
Cream	Fat-free half-and-half; fat-free nondairy creamer; fat-free evaporated milk
Eggs	Cholesterol-free egg substitutes; egg whites (2 for 1 whole egg)
Evaporated milk	Fat-free evaporated milk
Flavored salts, such as onion salt, garlic salt, and celery salt	Onion powder, garlic powder, celery seeds or flakes
Ice cream	Fat-free, low-fat, or light ice cream; fat-free or low-fat frozen yogurt; sorbet; sherbet; gelato
Salt	No-salt-added seasoning blends
Tomato juice	No-salt-added tomato juice
Tomato sauce	No-salt-added tomato sauce; 6-ounce can of no-salt-added tomato paste diluted with 1 can of water
Unsweetened baking chocolate	3 tablespoons cocoa powder plus 1 tablespoon unsaturated oil or light tub margarine for every 1-ounce square of chocolate
Whipping cream for topping	Fat-free whipped topping; fat-free evaporated milk (thoroughly chilled before whipping)
Whole milk	Fat-free milk

EMERGENCY SUBSTITUTIONS

When you see a recipe you'd like to prepare but don't have certain
ingredients on hand, or you begin a recipe only to find you're out of
something, try these in-a-pinch substitutions.

IF YOUR RECIPE CALLS FOR	USE
Allspice, 1 teaspoon	½ teaspoon ground cinnamon + 1 teaspoon ground cloves
Baking powder, 1 teaspoon	¼ teaspoon baking soda + ¾ teaspoon cream of tartar
Brown sugar, 1 cup	1 cup granulated sugar + 2 tablespoons molasses
Buttermilk, 1 cup	1 tablespoon vinegar or lemon juice + enough fat-free milk to equal 1 cup; or 1 cup fat-free plain yogurt
Cake flour, 1 cup sifted	1 cup minus 2 tablespoons sifted all-purpose flour
Confectioners' sugar, 1 cup	½ cup + 1 tablespoon granulated sugar
Cornstarch, 1 tablespoon	2 tablespoons all-purpose flour
Cracker crumbs, ¾ cup	¾ to 1 cup dry bread crumbs
Flour for thickening, 2 tablespoons all-purpose	1 tablespoon cornstarch
Flour, whole-wheat, 1 cup (for baking)	⅞ cup all-purpose flour
Fresh herbs, 1 tablespoon	1 teaspoon dried herbs
Gingerroot, peeled and grated, 1 tablespoon	⅛ teaspoon ground ginger
Honey, 1 tablespoon	1 tablespoon plus 1 teaspoon granulated sugar + 1½ teaspoons water
Lemon juice, 1 teaspoon	½ teaspoon vinegar
Lemon zest, 1 teaspoon	½ teaspoon lemon extract
Lemongrass	Grated lemon zest moistened with lemon juice
Onion, 1 small	1 teaspoon onion powder or 1 tablespoon minced dried onion
Ricotta cheese, ½ cup fat-free	½ cup fat-free cottage cheese

IF YOUR RECIPE CALLS FOR	USE
Sherry, 2 tablespoons	1 to 2 teaspoons vanilla extract
Sour cream, 1 cup fat-free	1 cup fat-free plain yogurt
Tomato juice, 1 cup	½ cup no-salt-added tomato sauce + ½ cup water
Tomato sauce, 2 cups	¾ cup no-salt-added tomato paste + 1 cup water
Wine, red, ½ cup	½ cup fat-free, no-salt-added beef broth or 1 tablespoon balsamic vinegar
Wine, white, ½ cup	½ cup fat-free, low-sodium chicken broth
Yeast, active dry, 1¼-ounce package	⅔ ounce cake yeast, crumbled

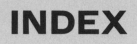

INDEX

salads (*continued*)

Spring Greens with Fruit, Goat Cheese, and Cranberry-Orange Vinaigrette, 74

Summer Pasta Salad, 81

Tomato-Artichoke Toss, 77

Tropical Tuna Salad, 90

salmon

fresh, cook's tip on, 109

Grilled Salmon Fillet with Fresh Herbs, 113

Salmon, Potatoes, and Green Beans en Papillote, 110–111

Salmon and Cucumber Salad with Basil-Lime Dressing, 89

Salmon with Mexican Rub and Chipotle Sour Cream Sauce, 112

Wine-Poached Salmon, 109

salsa

Pineapple-Kiwi Salsa, 270

Roasted Tomato Chipotle Salsa, 269

salt

substitutions for, 19, 24, 329

see also sodium

saturated fats, foods high in, 11, 17

sauces

Barbecue Sauce, 265

Chili Sauce, 276

Cinnamon Blueberry Sauce, 267

Gourmet Mushroom Sauce, 262

Spaghetti Sauce, 264

Strawberry Orange Sauce, 266–267

White Sauce, 260–261

White Sauce with Dijon Mustard, 261

White Sauce with Parmesan Cheese, 261

Yogurt Dill Sauce, 263

Sausage, Turkey, Patties, 166

Sautéed Trout with Cucumber-Melon Salsa, 120

savory, cook's tip on, 191

Scalloped Potatoes, 249

scallops

cook's tip on, 131

Scallops and Bok Choy with Balsamic Sauce, 130–131

seafood. *See* fish; shellfish

Seared Chicken with Fresh Pineapple, Ginger, and Mint Salsa, 135

seasonings

Chili Powder, 277

chili powder, cook's tip on, 190

Creole Seasoning, 278

jerk, cook's tip on, 195

low-salt substitution for, 329

no-sodium seasoning guide, 321

shopping guidelines, 19

seeds

dry-roasting, cook's tip on, 40

health benefits, 9

recommended daily servings, 323

shopping guidelines, 17

see also sesame seeds

sesame oil, cook's tip on, 94

sesame seeds

Grilled Sesame Chicken, 150

Sesame-Ginger Dressing, 95

shellfish

cook's tip on scallops, 131

Risotto with Shrimp and Vegetables, 128–129

Scallops and Bok Choy with Balsamic Sauce, 130–131

seasoning guide, 321

Shrimp and Spinach Pasta, 127

Spanish-Style Crab and Vegetable Tortilla, 132

shopping strategies

choosing from major food groups, 14–18

food packaging heart-check marks, 23

reading nutrition facts panel, 20–22

shrimp

Risotto with Shrimp and Vegetables, 128–129

Shrimp and Spinach Pasta, 127

side dishes

Asian Fried Rice with Peas, 253

Baked Beans, 238

Baked Italian Vegetable Mélange, 258

Balsamic Beets and Walnuts, 234–235

Barley and Chard Pilaf, 233

Brussels Sprouts with Caramelized Onions and Fennel, 240

Bulgur Pilaf with Kale and Tomatoes, 241

Citrus and Mint Quinoa with Feta Crumbles, 251

Creamy Carrots with Pecans, 242

Dilled Summer Squash, 256

Eggplant Mexicana, 244

Green Beans and Corn, 236–237

Greens with Tomatoes and Parmesan, 245

Orange-Glazed Butternut Squash, 255

Parmesan-Lemon Spinach, 254

Rice and Vegetable Pilaf, 252

Roasted Broccoli with Onions, 239

Roasted Plums with Walnut Crunch, 246–247

Roasted Red Peppers and Portobello Mushrooms, 248

Scalloped Potatoes, 249

Succotash, 237

Sweet Potato Casserole, 257

Tangy Roasted Asparagus, 232

Thyme-Flavored Cauliflower, 243

Zesty Oven-Fried Potatoes, 250

Sirloin with Red Wine and Mushroom Sauce, 175

Sirloin with Tomato, Olive, and Feta Topping, 178

Sliced Mango with Creamy Orange Sauce, 79

Slow-Cooker Beef and Red Beans, 188–189

Slow-Cooker Moroccan Chicken with Orange Couscous, 154–155

slow-cooking techniques, 26, 27

Smoked-Paprika Tuna Steaks with Spinach, 122–123

smoking, quitting, 32

Smoothies, Paradise, 296

snapper

Cajun Snapper, 115

Oregano Snapper with Lemon, 114

sodium

American Heart Association recommendations on, 2

average daily consumption, 1

common high-sodium foods, 324–325

compounds, types of, 22

dietary sources of, 6, 10, 324–325

on food labels, 22

health risks from, 2, 4–5

how to reduce in diet, 3, 6, 12–13, 14–19, 20–23, 24–29

My Sodium Tracker worksheet, 320

no-sodium seasoning guide, 321

in restaurant meals, 12–13

sole

Herbed Fillet of Sole, 118

Sole with Vegetables and Dijon Dill Sauce, 116–117